Health and Beauty from the Sea

ALSO BY THE SAME AUTHOR

How to Manage Your Man and Your Money

Health and Beauty from the Sea

By Molly Castle

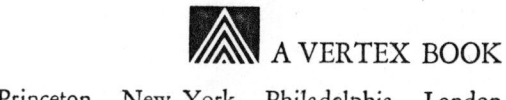 A VERTEX BOOK

Princeton   New York   Philadelphia   London

© Molly Castle, 1967

First published in USA 1971 by AUERBACH Publishers Inc.
by arrangement with Leslie Frewin Publishers Limited

Library of Congress Card Catalog No. 74-141790
ISBN 0-87769-064-2

Printed in the United States of America

DEDICATION:
Fame again

Contents

The Sea: What's in It for You	11
The Secret of Life	20
Eat Seaweed and Live to be 200	43
The Sunshine in Oil	65
The Sea Dwellers	93
Fish for Your Health	114
Breathe Deeper—Live Longer	136
Slim the Mermaid Way	151

Health and Beauty from the Sea

The Sea: What's in It for You

YOU MAY not want to live forever, but you would be unusual if you did not want to feel younger, be healthier and slimmer, and have a more pleasing appearance. Well, naturally. If I were to tell you that you could get all of these benefits right out of the sea, you probably would not believe me. That's exactly why I'm writing this book: just to prove it to you.

Most people feel that we haven't even begun to tap the sea's resources. This is certainly reassuring when you think how nearly used up the land is getting to be. For instance, there is the soil. It isn't only that it is being overused and undernourished; it is actually leaching away as well. Rain and floods, aided by wind, gravity, lightning, fires, and decay, carry topsoil into the ocean. With this topsoil go the minerals that should be in our plants, our food, animals and, eventually, in us. They are all in the sea, waiting to be reclaimed.

Minerals have been important to all our vital processes ever since life was first born in the sea from a chemical reaction in a water solution of all the minerals. They are truly essential to life.

Of course, even if the soil is impoverished, you won't go without minerals altogether. Except for iodine, which is found only in or near the sea, you may get in your land food *almost* enough minerals to be *almost* healthy.

Almost, though, isn't quite good enough. Why should we have to put up with all sorts of assorted little aches and pains, headaches, sleeplessness, poor teeth and bones, colds in winter, lassitude in summer—all this and overweight too?

Besides, there's the iodine which is not naturally in any land food (it can, of course, be added, as is the case with iodized salt). But originally it comes only from the sea.

Iodine, which you may think of in terms of a small bottle of disinfectant which you dab on cuts, is enormously important to our health and well-being. Without enough of it, the gland which governs the rate at which we burn our food cannot function. Without about enough to balance on the head of a pin we would be as brainless as vegetables and not half as useful. Animals and vegetables from the sea contain this mineral. It is vital to health and beauty.

But back to the salt mines. The most common ingredient of seawater—salt—is a necessity to all living creatures. It controls the balance of liquids in the tissues; our bodies, like those of other animals, are about seventy-five percent water.

What land food hasn't lost from the soil has been lost in the refinery. Says one doctor: "Super-refinement of natural foodstuffs has probably been as successful in promoting ill-health in the past two generations as the most virulent of disease germs."

Seafood is not tampered with; the minerals it is supposed to have, it has—in full supply. Seawater, sea plants, and every kind of fish contain them. Feeding in their rich marine pasture, fish can always get the maximum of vital food elements and pass them on to us. Cows, pigs, sheep, poultry are, in this respect, as unreliable as the land from which they feed. This land may be largely depleted of the minerals that should be in it.

Yet we eat from six to ten times more meat and poultry than fish—which is sad as well as uneconomical. For the land animals will rarely contain, on the dinner table, the amount of minerals attributed to them in the nutrition tables.

There's something else important, too: protein, which means "of first importance." The flesh of fish, like our own, is composed largely of protein, And not only our flesh but also our skin, hair, nails. For that matter, so are our brains not to mention our eyes, ears, legs, sex appeal— the lot. Protein is the most basic ingredient of every part of our body. It is also needed for repair jobs. If parts of us break down and need an overhaul, the repair is going to get done one way or another; but if it is carried out with straw instead of bricks, it isn't going to be a very good job and it isn't going to last.

Of course, we can get protein by eating beef, lamb, pork, poultry, dairy products and some vegetables. But meat is more expensive than fish and has a kind of fat which can be harmful; for those who are dieting (and who isn't?) most servings of meat have twice the calories of an equivalent serving of fish and as much as four times that of shellfish.

The trouble with us is we are rather conservative. We eat very few kinds of fish and cook them in a rather prosaic and unimaginative fashion—rarely to their best advantage. There are many varieties we scarcely even try. Skate, for instance. Skate appears on the menus of most expensive restaurants under the title *raie au beurre,* but fish markets seldom stock it and can still more rarely sell it if they do. I don't know what we would make of pompano; we think octopus, like frogs' legs, is strictly for the French. And caviar is for the wealthy, although there are many tasty fish eggs at lower prices.

We boil cod, fry flounder, coat whiting in fattening batter; we eat pilchards and sardines only from cans, never attempt whitebait at all. Well, I've been collecting some fabulous recipes for making any fish you can eat exciting, even on a slimming diet.

We live our lives feeling guilt because we are overweight. Our part of the world is eating too much; we feel guilty, too, that the rest of the world isn't eating enough.

What is coming to be called aquaculture has the answer: lower-calorie food for ourselves, higher-protein food for those exploding populations. There is more than enough foodstuff in the oceans of the world.

I read in a nutrition magazine that the richer countries eat as much as sixty grams of protein a day. In India they only average six. This, said the magazine—which is, of course, why I'm quoting it—could be solved by using the so-far poorly tapped source of food in the ocean. "More fish," it suggested, "could be made into meal to be given to animals. The animals could then be eaten by human beings."

Or why not eat the fish direct?

There are two other sources of food in the sea: algae and plankton. Plankton are the wanderers on the surface of the sea; they have no means of locomotion. They are either plant or animal, and are so small that thousands of them would fit into a teaspoon. A way has now been found to turn them into various types of food, for they are extremely nourishing and well-balanced nutritionally. The Japanese make soup cubes of plankton. It makes excellent fish paste. More and more ways of using it are being researched. There is enough of it in the sea to feed a population exploding into outer space.

Then there is marine algae, a polite way of saying seaweed. Far from being weeds, sea algae have remarkable health and beauty properties. Liquid seaweed, used on land plants, provides them with every mineral they need to turn them into healthy, vitamin-rich food. As a food supplement seaweed tablets are very beneficial. For one thing, they feed the thyroid gland, providing a special ingredient for the manufacture of its hormone, thyroxin. This hormone regulates the way our food burns. Remember, a slow-burning digestive system leaves behind it unused food which nestles onto various parts of us as nasty little rolls of fat.

Marine algae can be slimming in another way: in baths. Some models who could qualify as mermaids if they only had fish tails, swear by marine algae baths. They open the pores of the skin, encourage sweating, remove waste products, many of a fatty nature, and substitute good sea minerals in their place.

Talking of models, have you noticed that they are never overweight? This may be due to their low-calorie fish diet or it may be due to the fact that they swim a good deal. A model I once met told me about some out-of-this-world exercises that she and her sisters practice. In due course I will pass the secret on to you.

Models, too, probably know of a few oils from the sea that can make them beautiful: cod liver oil, halibut liver oil, shark oil, turtle and some others, even the oils from herring, mackerel and other of the so-called fat fish (well, they may be fat, but they are never obese).

As you well know, some kinds of fats—animal fats, solid fats—can be bad for you. Not only your figure but also your arteries and your heart suffer from too much of this solid animal fat. Yet a certain type and amount of fat is essential to life, as necessary as the other vital ingredients we've talked about. Two of these elements are so important that they are known as the essential fatty acids—EFA for short. The fat fishes contain these, and fish livers are the very best known source in existence.

One reason that some fat is essential is that without it we could not make use of certain vitamins—those known as "fat-soluble." These are vitamins A, the skin and eye vitamin; D, the one needed for strong bones; and E, the reproductive processes' standby. Naturally, all three of these are needed for beauty as well as health.

Bones, for instance. Good bone structure is part of a beautiful body. You can't be very healthy if your bones keep breaking up. Without an adequate supply of vitamin D children get rickets and adults develop brittle bones.

Vitamin D is not an easy vitamin to come by. It is derived from sunshine—which is fine if you live in the Caribbean or California. It is also in the sea wanderers—plankton—which pick up the sun's rays and transform them into a life-giving substance. This vital ingredient is sometimes known as X: we don't know how to reproduce it. Some people think it is the essence of life itself.

Cod fish swallow plankton every time they open their big mouths, and they store the oil and the sunshine in their livers. When we take cod liver oil or capsules, we are getting the sunshine vitamin D equivalent of a holiday in Spain.

Ingredient X is now thought to be the reason why cod liver oil prevents and even cures tuberculosis (now once again on the increase), why it is lethal to certain of the more unpleasant bacteria—for instance, streptococcus, which causes septic (or "strep"), throat; staphlylococcus, known as the hospital "bug" because it can devastate an entire hospital; and pneumococcus, responsible for some types of pneumonia.

Jersey cows—those that still live in Guernsey in the Channel Islands—are free from tuberculosis. These cows wander along the seashore munching on sea plants that have been washed by waves containing, one assumes, the mysterious ingredient X. These cows are also free from reproductive disasters. Primitive people, living far inland, make expeditions to the shore to bring back seaweed which they dry and give to their marriageable girls. This duty falls to Maori mothers-in-law who walk three hundred miles over mountains so that they will have healthy grandchildren. Modern mothers-in-law save themselves a lot of walking by just going down to the clinic and getting a bottle of cod liver oil. They take it themselves, too, if they have arthritis. It's a folk medicine remedy with which science has finally caught up.

A rich and constant source of vitamin A is halibut oil. Not only is vitamin A essential for healthy skins, but the eyes need it also. As with minerals, in sea vitamins you can always get what you count on. Land products analyzed for their vitamin content vary widely. The quantities assessed them are usually maximum because the products analyzed come from good soil and are grown under the best of conditions. Test vegetables may even contain up to a hundred times more vitamin A than those which have grown on poor, depleted soil, traveled long distances, suffered from storing, canning, cooking. But the "soil" of the sea is never overworked or underfed, as a market garden on land can be.

But it isn't only the oils from the sea that you swallow

that benefit your skin. Several fish oils are remarkable in the effect they have when you use them in beauty creams.

Not long ago a French cosmetic chemist set out to discover what kind of oil would penetrate deepest through the top layer of the skin. An oil which would sink right down to the skin's lowest level, he reasoned (skin is rather like an onion; it has layers), would be an invaluable medium for transporting to where they would do the most good, certain rejuvenating serums he had discovered. It is on this basement level that wrinkles are formed and skin toughens and dries up. He colored a number of different oils, including some old standbys like lanolin, coconut oil, vaseline, but none of them did just what he wanted them to do. Tracing the course of the various colored oils on the skin of a test animal, he was amazed to find that shark oil proved to have by far the greatest penetration. This made it a first-class medium for those biological miracles that he wanted to send down to the living cells where they could wipe out wrinkles and about ten years.

This shark oil is now known as Perydrosqualene—goodness knows why, unless it is just to make things difficult. A shark by any other name—in fact any type of shark—does equally well, since all sharks have a considerable quantity of fat immediately beneath their skin. This fat is melted and distilled. The end product is colorless and nongreasy and never goes rancid.

The French cosmetologist is also very impressed with the properties of turtle oil. He believes it to be the only oil which is both a softener and an astringent. This, he says, makes it ideal for the skin around the eyes—some creams, as you may know to your cost, cause puffiness. Turtle oil never does.

They do say that Cleopatra used turtle oil and that

was how she came to look like Elizabeth Taylor. Get some and you too can look like Elizabeth Taylor—unless it would be more appropriate for you to look like Richard Burton. Well, he probably borrows her soap. Turtle oil soap produces a fine rich penetrating lather which moisturizes rather than dries.

Every year, every day probably, more and more valuable discoveries are made—and I don't mean just that there is gold, oil, diamonds and such under the waves. For instance, doctors say that there are as many, or more antibiotics as on land; there's a conch oil which may soon be of inestimable value in arthritis; seaweed has been found to destroy some of the evil by products of atomic waste, and it has also proved effective in oxidizing the air and removing carbon dioxide in submarines and space ships—which may be a very important discovery indeed.

As I said in the beginning, the sea is crammed full of a rich harvest of beauty, health, youth.

Be my guest—dive in . . . .

The Secret of Life

SEAWATER. Well, first of all there's an awful lot of it. It occupies more than seventy percent of the earth's surface. It's a good thing it doesn't cover any more. If at some date the climate of the earth changed and the ice at the Poles melted, the waters of the oceans would cover the eastern seaboard of the United States, most of England and Europe and goodness knows how many other places. As it is, however, the sea is potentially, historically and actually a source of life. We couldn't do without it.

From the ocean all life started. In the sea, in the waters of the sea, is the secret of life itself. Scientists know it is there although they have never quite been able to capture it. One scientist reconstructed seawater with all its chemical components in exact ratio. Into a jar of this he set some sea plants to grow. They would not live, he discovered, unless he added a small quota of real seawater in which, he was obliged to assume, was an ingredient he had been unable to reproduce.

Of course, the oceans have been rich with minerals since the beginning of time—time itself has only added to them.

The first big rainfall on earth—the flood—was a very long time before Noah or any other human being. They say the rain fell for hundreds of years. Probably there was no water before that. The earth itself was made from molten star dust that had got caught up in orbit round the sun, gradually cooled off and cracked, so that mountains and valleys were formed.

When the rain began to fall in torrents it gradually filled up all the crevices, cracks and hollows. Water rushed down the mountain sides carrying, even then, salts and chemicals, lava and broken rock. Every chemical and mineral that arrived from outer space, every little bit of star dust, dropped its quota into the ocean. Some parts of these dissolved, others sank below the surface. Some scientists say that in the very core of the earth, beneath the waters, there is still molten iron. At a much more practical depth, waiting to be unearthed (or rather unsea'd), are all the minerals and oils and ores and coal that we could possibly want for centuries to come.

Rains still fall and wear away the hills and the mountains. Floods carry the topsoil of the valleys into the rivers. The earth's store of minerals is gradually being depleted and washed into the ocean. Glaciers gather all before them and when, in the course of time, they become icebergs, they gradually melt and add their quota of the earth's valuables to those already in the depths.

All the minerals dug from the earth and made into motor cars, pots and pans, washing machines and houses gradually corrode, find their way to rubbish heaps. These, too, are eventually washed away.

Gasoline, coal and wood are burned, the smoke goes into the air, where it is caught by clouds and deposited by rain, much of it on to the seas. The air itself has, in any case, always been a potential lifegiver to water, containing as it does, soluble vital elements such as oxygen, carbon, hydrogen and nitrogen.

Modern sanitation, meteors from outer space, underwater upheavals, man-made upheavals (wars and the products thereof) have all aided in making the sea a repository for much of the mineral wealth once in the land.

At this point of time they do say that there are fifty quadrillion tons of dissolved mineral salts in the oceans of the world. Clearly if we could get some of them back, there would be more than enough to go around.

It was a comparatively short time ago, historically and medically speaking—perhaps about twenty years ago—that a new enemy appeared on the nutrition horizon: mineral deficiency.

The new enemy was a negative not a positive thing like, say, a germ of a virus. It was, in itself, an incompleteness, a lack of something that should have been in the soil but which had been either used up or washed out.

Plants grown on mineral-poor soil may look all right. They may be green and apparently flourishing. But they have much less food value. Furthermore, if the soil is both leached of minerals by excessive rainfall and fatigued by overcultivation, the plants get poorer and poorer in quality and quantity each year. Without the right minerals in their correct proportions plants do not produce the vitamins that they should have. Food animals fed from poor soil or on plants grown in poor soil are not up to standard either.

In 1945, Dr. William Albrecht, a leader in soil chemistry, said: "Doctors, through experiment and observation in nutritional research, have begun to understand that many diseases can be traced to dietary deficiencies and that many sick people are hungry people. People can eat three square meals a day and still suffer from deficiencies. One of these hidden hungers is for calcium, another for iron, copper, cobalt, iodine, zinc and so on."

Minerals, of course, are essential to life. We must have iron in our blood; its function is to utilize the oxygen which we breathe from the air. We need also a trace of copper; without copper, iron cannot be assimilated. Bones, and many other parts of us, are made from or with calcium. The thyroid gland needs not only iodine but also a trace of zinc. Could you have guessed—unless you already knew—that tonsillitis is associated with a deficiency of silver? Phosphorus combines with calcium to make bones and teeth and is needed in the soft tissues of the body. These also help the blood to clot and assure that muscles and nerves react normally. Iron, with its assistant, copper, is involved with protein in making red blood cells. As well as calcium and phosphorus, teeth need another mineral, fluorine, to help them resist decay. Certain of the vitamins need certain of the minerals before they can be effectively utilized. For instance, B12 was recognized fairly recently to require iron and copper before it could help in the creation of healthy blood, and B12 also has a mineral ingredient: cobalt.

Vitamin D is associated with calcium and phosphorus in bone building and with silicon in the manufacture of hair and nails. The chain is endless and interreacting. It is also admitted by scientists that foods almost certainly contain other important ingredients that have not yet been recognized individually.

There are around three hundred and thirty million cubic miles of seawater. Its best-known ingredient is salt. Salt is a mineral. It is also a taste. People sailed the seas searching for this taste hundreds of years ago. In those days, before refrigerators, salt was also widely used as a preservative of fish and meat. Nature—or who else?—gave us the taste for salt because it is a necessary ingredient of our bodies. Blood, sweat and tears need salt for their composition.

The mineral in seawater which gives it its taste is sodium chloride, which accounts for eighty-five percent of sea salt. The most important function of this mineral is to regulate the distribution of water in our tissues; in this capacity it enters into the composition of every fluid in us. It has a great affinity for water, as you must have found out if you have ever left a salt cellar around in damp weather. Without it our tissues dry out. One enterprising cosmetician has discovered that the secret of the sea, at least as far as moisturizing the skin goes, is salt: sodium chloride, in fact. Outside the skin, as well as underneath, the salt attracts moisture.

Our taste for salt is given us because we must have it for regulating internal secretions. It's the same thing with animals. If deprived of salt, cattle will search everywhere for a salt lick.

In tropical countries or in competitive sports, where loss of salt through sweating is frequent, faintness, cramps and other symptoms are relieved by salt tablets. Olympic athletes have had to retire with cramp if they haven't prepared themselves for this loss. In some countries salt has even become a political issue—remember Gandhi's salt marches?

There is a belief that salt makes people fat. Well, it can make them appear fat—or rather bloated. If they have taken in more salt than they can use or excrete, it may attract water and retain it in the tissues. This is known as edema. It can be eliminated by exercise, Turkish baths, diuretics, etc. These will get rid of the excess fluid and will cause a weight loss. But it will be water that will have been lost, not fat.

We need five grams a day which, of course, is practically impossible to measure. Salt is added to processed foods, found naturally in meat and fish and usually eaten in butter and cheese. Too much is said to be bad for the arteries but how much is too much? An egg without salt is like a kiss without a moustache.

I don't know where the legend started that seawater will make one mad. Perhaps the conditions in which one might find oneself with water, water everywhere and not a drop to drink would be conducive to madness. Being on an open raft, say, under a pitiless sun and with little chance of rescue would be enough to drive anyone round the bend. And althought salt water, in itself, can't really affect the mind, it is not thirst quenching, and prolonged thirst can make people crazy. But in small quantities, as well as, not instead of, fresh water, it will kill all known germs. Animals and primitive men, in whom instinct is still active, try to bathe wounds in the ocean. Medical men today are recommending sea bathing for fracture cases, arthritis, skin diseases and other conditions.

In 1963 a seventy-year-old man sailed across the Pacific alone on a raft. He reported after finding himself with various bodily discomforts: "I began to realise that I must do something about my body. And I knew what to do. Each morning at dawn I daubed salt water on my eyes to relieve the burning from the sun; I splashed seawater on my face and I inhaled it, for it cleared the nasal passages. Then I drank one mug of seawater every day to counteract the sun's dehydrating effect. Believe me, seawater has medicinal powers. It must have for my body cured."

There is a legend among beauty editors that seawater is bad for the hair. Nothing could be further from the truth, as any responsible hairdresser will tell you. After sea bathing it should be allowed to dry on but not in the full sunlight; it is the sun not the salt water which does the damage. The salt water can be showered off later if the hair feels sticky. Personally I have found that the seawater gives the hair so much body that my hair (if it has been well cut) does not even need to be set at the hairdresser's—just combed through and pushed into place.

If you put a saucer full of seawater into a flat dish and heat it in the oven, or under a strong sun, the water will dry out and white powdery crystals will remain. This is, of course, sea salt. Eighty-five percent of it will be sodium chloride—salty tasting—and the rest will be the other minerals. Most of these are trace minerals, so-called because the quantity of each is so small you can barely see it through a microscope. Yet they are so essential to the workings of our body that without them illness and death could result.

In its natural state all foodstuffs come complete with all the ingredients arranged in the proportion in which we need them. When we start removing various elements to make foods taste better, last longer, look prettier or, in the case of salt, pour more easily, we are destroying a good deal of their value. Sea salt contains just those minerals we have in our bloodstream and in the correct ratio. Table salt has had most of them removed. Indeed one can hardly buy sea salt—that is, whole and intact—except in a health store. Table salt, however, usually has at least one sea mineral replaced. This is iodine.

If you can't get untampered-with sea salt, then at least be sure to get the iodized version, and nobody should give up salt altogether except under doctors' orders. These are only given when something has gone wrong with the water-distributing system of the body. If this is working normally, as it is with nearly everybody, too little salt will, as with the athletes, just give you cramp.

Iodine is the one mineral that comes only from the sea. It is not found in the land unless that land is near enough to the sea to have been watered by salt spray. In 1882 a French doctor realized that iodine deficiency brought about many disturbances of the body and particularly was a cause of goiter. He had noticed that this unpleasant illness, one symptom of which is the marked swelling of the throat, occurred in inland places where there was no iodine in the soil. He was advanced enough to suggest iodizing table salt which, even in those days, must have been "purified," since iodine is an ingredient of natural salt. But it took fifty years and thousands of goiter sufferers before the idea became generally accepted.

Sea spray, so fine it cannot be seen, or so thick that it is called mist or fog, can penetrate some distance. In a small country like England there are not too many counties so far removed from the effects of sea spray that there is no iodine at all in the soil. In larger continents iodine shortage can be acute. There are "goiter belts" even now in some inland parts of the United States and in inland countries like Switzerland, though with improved transportation and refrigeration seafood can be obtained far inland and, besides that, the French doctor's eighty-year-old suggestion has now been widely accepted.

The reason a deficiency of iodine causes a swelling in the neck is because the thyroid gland in the throat needs this mineral to form its hormone, thyroxin. As you know, each of the endocrine glands manufactures its own special hormone which acts as its messenger. When a gland needs something, it sends its errand boy to alert the other parts of the body. The thyroid gland uses its messenger, among other things, to organize the burning (or metabolizing or digesting, whichever you like to call it) of everything we eat.

If not enough iodine is forthcoming, the gland works overtime trying to extract enough from too much inanimate material and it leaves behind a sort of slag heap of rubbish sitting untidily in the front of the neck. Even though it works overtime, it still may not get sufficient iodine for an adequate supply of thyroxin. People with too little of this hormone in the blood and tissues burn their food too slowly and store too much of it as fat.

Most of the symptoms of deficiency can be relieved by the addition of iodine to the diet but some effects, if the shortage has continued too long, may be irreversible. One of these is a pressure on the eyeballs. Another may be an inability to have children. Prevention is far better because the thyroid gland requires iodine for other purposes. The brain needs it. Sluggishness, as well as overweight, is a symptom of iodine shortage. Iodine also kills harmful germs in the bloodstream—in the same manner as it disinfects cuts and wounds on the outside. Our blood passes through the thyroid once every seventeen minutes for just this purpose.

In certain cases of accident to the thyroid gland iodine is not enough. If the gland is severely damaged due to some misadventure and is unable to manufacture its hormone, thyroxin has to be administered direct.

I heard of a boy who had been in a car accident which had cut his throat and obliterated the thyroid gland. The throat, of course, was repaired along with many other damaged areas, but the loss of the gland was not immediately recognized. But from being a bright child he became dull and retarded. He gained weight but he was mentally and physically comatose. Brain damage was suspected until one expert diagnostician realized what must have happened and put the boy on a course of thyroxin. Very soon he started to improve. By the time he reached his teens he was a brilliant student, but the relatives with whom he lived—his parents had been killed in the accident—failed to warn him of the absolute necessity of his daily pill. The routine bored him and, on holiday, he gave it up. Very gradually he began to regress. After a few weeks he became almost childish and eventually slipped back into near imbecility. Then, fortunately, the cause was again recognized and he was restored to normal by the renewed administration of his daily dose.

This, of course, is an exaggerated case. Most people keep their thyroid intact, more or less. No accident eliminates it. But even a mild shortage of iodine over a long period can have a bad effect. Overweight can stem from a sluggish metabolism when food is burned too slowly. A tendency to colds and other infections, to enlarged adenoids, to a generalized fatigue, to a lack of joy in living, can all be indications.

One of the important jobs of the thyroid gland and one for which it needs iodine is to keep hair young and strong. It is because there is so much of this in the diet of the Aran Islanders, who live by and from the sea, that their hair remains thick and black until a late age.

Iodine, in fact, also helps to retard other symptoms of ageing. Dr. Ward Crampton said in a booklet *Live Long and Like It*: "Iodine poverty is a common accompaniment of ageing after the fortieth year. The basic requirement is only 0.2 milligrams daily. Yet an active but over-tired man of fifty, with a thyroid deficiency, may get as much stimulation and far more real benefit from a few milligrams of iodine than from a cocktail."

Tiny though it is, the thyroid gland is of enormous importance to health and well-being. If you want proof of this, you can get it from the fact that the rate of blood flowing through it is about twenty-five percent greater than the rate of blood flowing through the kidneys and about forty percent greater than that through the lungs.

The engineer who invented the human body arranged it so because thyroxin is needed in great supply throughout every part of the body as an oxidizing agent: it supplies oxygen.

Mothers who receive sufficient iodine bear children who seldom have adenoids. As many primitive people traditionally realize, it is necessary for fertility.

Although iodine is the only mineral exclusive to the sea, the waters of the oceans contain, in full supply, all the other minerals which should be, but often are not, in the soil of the land. Still, even after nutrition researchers first recognized our need for minerals, they were not too worried that we would go short of them. With the exception of iodine they were all in the earth's soil, they reasoned. Therefore we should get enough of them by eating plants and animals that had fed from the soil . . . until people like Dr. Albrecht began to associate poor soil, impoverished soil, with poor health.

Since all the mineral elements that are needed to make us healthy—or to put it more strongly, to prevent us getting ill—should be in the soil it doesn't take much imagination to appreciate what happens when the soil no longer contains them. But it does take imagination as well as expert knowledge sometimes to detect which element is lacking. There was a doctor in Monmouthshire, England, for example, who made a quite brilliant deduction. His patient was the small daughter of a local farmer: a pale, sickly, anemic child who slept badly, had a poor appetite and had a peculiar habit which very much distressed her mother: she was a dirt eater. From the time the little girl could crawl she had scooped up handfuls of earth and chewed them up. Indoors she took the soil from potted plants.

The doctor realized, of course, that this was the child's need to compensate for something lacking in her food—but what? Calcium? That seemed a possibility but she got plenty of milk and dairy produce to give her enough calcium and phosphorus, as well as the sunshine vitamin D these need for their utilization. Iron and/or copper? He had the local soil analyzed and there was no shortage of these. Then he went back to the milk and decided to investigate the herd of cows from which the milk came.

He had read that in some parts of the world—Australia, for one, and in some areas of the United States—cows were dying of a crippling form of anemia. It had been discovered that this was due to deficiency of cobalt and could be prevented when a few pounds of cobalt were added to each acre of land.

He referred again to his soil analysis and found that this mineral was indeed deficient. The grass on which the cows were grazing, the milk and meat which they produced, the vegetables, chickens, eggs—everything grown on or feeding from the soil—was short in cobalt. It could not be otherwise.

It is now known, of course, that B12, of which cobalt is a constituent, is the factor in liver which cures and prevents simple anemia, and even pernicious anemia, because without it red blood cells will not form. Our doctor decided to try the child on a course of B12 while at the same time recommending to the farmer that he add cobalt to his land. Almost immediately she gave up chewing dirt. Soon she was sleeping and eating better. Within a month the child had improved beyond recognition.

You can't tell mineral-poor soil to look at it and it is not always possible to recognize mineral deficiencies in people. Yet, as with this child, there are often indications. Nail-biting may be one. Irritability, slow growth rate, anemia, mental apathy, poor bone and teeth formation, lack of energy, sleeplessness, may all show the need for a greater supply of minerals than is being obtained. So can premature ageing.

In Iran it was found that men who failed to develop or maintain sexual potency were suffering from a shortage of zinc. The gonads, or sex glands, also require iron. Other glands need other minerals. The pituitary uses chlorine and manganese, the adrenal glands require magnesium, the pancreas needs nickel and cobalt.

Even when all these and the rest of the vital minerals are in the soil, they may not be there in optimum quantities. Potassium in short supply in the soil can make animals slow in growth, nervous and disturbed and cause gas formation and constipation. All the minerals are in rich supply in sea water and in all food which is grown in it. Potassium, for instance, is closely related to sodium and chlorine—salt, that is—in regulating glandular secretions. Seawater is like soil in the sense that it is the medium of growth for growing or living things. Everything that comes from it can provide us with a wealth of health and beauty.

It is true that soil depleted and overworked can recoup itself if given time, but few farmers can afford to leave their lands idle. Ploughing back, or adding fertilizer, helps, especially a fertilizer which is derived from the sea and contains all the sea's wealth of minerals—a seaweed fertilizer, for instance, or one made from the droppings of birds who have fed from fish—guano. In Norway they add salt seawater to a chalky substance that, while now on land, was originally under the sea and, among all the other sea minerals, contains calcium from millions of crushed shells and fish bones. Soil so restored provides essential minerals in the correct, natural ratio in which they are needed by animals and people. Like the artificial seawater which would not sustain life, artificial fertilizers may be, and usually are, unbalanced and do not contain that mysterious essence of life which is so important, but a fertilizer derived from the sea contains the phosphates and nitrates that are needed for soil improvement.

Fertilizers and other chemical products are made from salts deposited in inland seas no longer—if they ever were—tidal. The Dead Sea is one of these. The Salton Sea in California is another. Where there are no tides, and evaporation from the sun takes place, the concentration of minerals in the water gradually strengthens. And now there is a new source. Ordinary seawater taken straight out of the sea is being used as a source not only of minerals but of fresh water as well.

In the summer of 1965 the Eastern seaboard of the United States was so dry that Americans even had to do without their ubiquitous glass of iced water with their meals. They were not allowed to water their gardens or even their window boxes. They were politely advised by the authorities that it was not really necessary to flush their toilets except for something serious. Even dishwashers suspended action. Many parts of the world depend for their water supply on a precarious rainfall: in Bermuda, for instance, there are neither wells nor rivers nor lakes of fresh water—rain is trapped on the roofs and guided into tanks. For large hotels with limited roof space and unlimited tourists this is not enough. In Southern California it only rains one or two months a year; some years it never rains at all in the Algarve, Portugal. In 1959, during a bad shortage, West Germany had to send fire engines around the villages selling water.

So naturally scientists have had to devise a suitable method for converting seawater, of which there is an unlimited supply. Various methods are used based more or less on the principle of distillation. It is an expensive way of getting fresh water. The bonus of minerals from the sea makes up for this.

Seawater can be used for many things; more ways are being discovered all the time. Other things are also being invented: unfortunately, in some aspects, atomic power, for instance. Like many things people on land want to discard, radioactive waste is now being dumped in the ocean. Happily, there is something in the sea which can counteract the effects to a great extent. We'll come to that later.

Many people, however, still fear that the vast volume of water will be contaminated by fall-out. "This possibility exists," says one scientific journal, "although the danger is negligible as compared with the hazards that now threaten our health from the use of land harvests. Virtually every acre of our agricultural crops, with very few exceptions, is contaminated, not only with fall-out but with poisonous chemicals which we are accumulating in the cells of our bodies."

"We can use to advantage," the article continues, "seawater itself, which seems to supply the trace mineral elements required as a dietary supplement. Seawater increases the assimiliation of vitamins, proteins and other nutrients. It has many values. For example, it can be added to the dough in bread-making to supply the minerals that have been extracted by processing methods."

This, of course, would have to be done on a rather wider scale than most householders can achieve. But by adding sea salt to vegetables as we cook them—or to any other food for that matter that needs salt—we can get the benefit of the valuable trace minerals not supplied by ordinary table salt and no longer to be safely counted as a natural part of vegetables.

The nutrition expert, the late Dr. Bircher-Benner of Zürich, Switzerland, said: "Sea salt, which contains minerals in their true balance, enhances and emphasises the natural taste of foods. Ordinary salt disguises it."

Minerals, obviously, are solvent in water or they wouldn't be in the sea water itself. Many vitamins are also water soluble. It is of little use to add sea salt to vegetable cooking and then pour the minerals it supplies down the drain. One manufacturer of vitamin-mineral supplements told me gleefully that the public (via its cooks) throws thousands of pounds worth of minerals and vitamins down the drain. The television doesn't help. In a lesson on expert vegetable cooking the water from every pan full of vegetables went down the drain with every housewife who had tuned in ready to do likewise; so do save the water and use it for stock.

Potassium—which you may remember is the mineral closely related to sodium and chlorine in the formation of blandular secretions—not only goes down the drain with the water but is also largely lost when food is refined. Nutritionist Adelle Davis says: "A partial deficiency of potassium in animals causes slow growth, constipation, gas formation, and a nervousness typified by extreme alertness and insomnia. The symptoms are so similar to those endured by millions of people that a study was made of human subjects maintained on a diet low in potassium. All developed constipation, indigestion, insomnia and nervousness. Our high consumption of refined foods and our sloppy cooking methods, to say nothing of the condition of our soil, could easily allow unrecognised potassium deficiency to be widespread."

This equally applies to all the other water-soluble minerals. These are to be found not only in seawater, but in all seafood, as we will see in later chapters.

BEAUTY FROM SEAWATER

SLIMMING

The sea, seawater, and much that it contains, as well as some special exercises that you can do in seawater, are so important for those who want to slim (and who doesn't?) that I have devoted a complete section to slimming exercises on page 162.

The sea mineral which is most important in slimming is iodine since it works directly for the gland which controls the rate at which we burn our food.

FINGERNAILS

Iodine is useful here, too. Choose a polish remover that contains it: it counteracts the harm that can be done by the acetone.

YOUTHFULNESS

The sea and its minerals can keep you young in many ways. Here are four of them:

1 By building resistance to disease. Ill health, whether of infectious or degenerative origin, is always aging.

2 By restoring, repairing, rebuilding worn-out tissues.

3 By aiding the glands to function fully.

4 By regulating the acid-alkali balance in the blood and tissues.

SKIN HEALTH

Sun and sunbathing can be beneficial in many ways but they have their dangers. But most sun-tan lotions and creams and jellies contain a filter to keep out the more harmful rays. There is one sun-tan jelly which contains just those sea salts that attract and hold water in the tissues thereby counteracting the drying effect of the sun's rays on the skin.

The disinfectant properties of seawater are excellent. It is valuable in many skin disorders and for cuts and wounds.

HEALTH FROM SEAWATER

Many people can get to the sea for only a few weeks a year, if at all. But everyone can benefit from its salts. Sea salt can be obtained from health stores, from many large shops or direct from the distributors. It comes either for the table or for the bath.

For a sore throat, a threatened cold or after being close to a source of any kind of respirtaory infection, dissolve a teaspoon of sea salt in boiling or very hot water then cool to blood heat. Gargle about once an hour, spit out and then swallow a fresh sip so that the salt is able to reach parts of the throat the gargle could not touch. Due to their affinity for water, sodium chloride and potassium help to dry up a runny nose and watery eyes.

It is the iodine in seawater—or sea salt—which is the chief disinfectant. It is the thyroid gland's iodine secretion which kills germs in the bloodstream: weak germs immediately and stronger ones after several passages of the blood through the thyroid.

Iodine can also kill germs on the outside of the body. You probably remember that dark brown stuff which your grandmother used to put on your cuts. Iodine, in solution, can now be bought decolorized. Buy it in a bottle which has a plastic applicator. It can be painted onto infected gums and as well as helping the outside of the gums, will be absorbed into the bloodstream to help kill the underlying infection. It is a healer as well as a disinfectant.

One drop of iodine solution in an acid drink—such as fruit juice—reduces tension, irritability and even sleeplessness.

Although we need very little, we can still get too little even if our food appears to supply it. Chlorine and sometimes fluorine, used to disinfect tap water, can displace iodine by a law of chemistry known as halogen displacement. To replace this, it is not necessary to take more than one drop twice a week. Yet although so little is needed, it is vital to health.

SEAWATER AND ARTHRITIS

Arthritis is a complex condition which is largely due to the fact that the human body, like all engines, wears out in time. But since not everybody gets it, it is not an essential part of old age. It may prove something if a certain group of people have lived for centuries on a certain type of diet and never had arthritis. Or it may not; perhaps it was their climate. A dry, warm, equable climate is perhaps the answer. Nevertheless I had a letter from a waggish friend of mine who said: "I came to the desert for arthritis and I got it." So even the climate isn't always the deciding factor.

Some people say that exercise is the thing. People who have exercised a great deal in youth and then given it up often get it, they claim. Indians who have done Yogi exercises all their lives never do. But the diets of these two groups may also have some relevance. Former sportsmen who once watched their weight, exercised away any excess, now may eat and drink more, take less care and perhaps take no exercise at all. Increased weight on the weight-bearing joints can't help being a factor in wearing them down.

This is where exercise may help both in shedding weight and limbering up stiff joints. This is particularly so when these exercises are done in salt water since water is buoyant and supports the weight of the body while the movements are being carried out. Furthermore, there is a bonus from the chemical salts in seawater which in themselves can be absorbed through the skin and of these iodine is particularly helpful.

Swimming in the ocean is one of the most valuable of all arthritis exercises. It is certainly nonweight bearing—try floating around your bedroom three feet from the ground. Swimming can exercise painful joints without being painful. Even lying in the surf at the water's edge and letting the waves surge over you is excellent for the circulation and therefore is beneficial. It helps the system remove the small particles of bone that the disease may have dislodged and it tends to prevent cramp.

However, few people live where they can swim all the year round in the ocean. Most of us manage no more than a couple of weeks. A good deal can be done right in your own bathtub, especially if you first convert it to salt seawater by the addition of sea salt.

Get the bathwater at the right temperature—almost, but not quite, too hot. Pour in the sea salt, preferably first melted down in very hot water. Provide yourself with a bath pillow; these are covered in plastic and fitted with rubber suction cups. If you are a person who can't remember exercises unless you see them written down, you had better also provide yourself with a chair on which to prop this book, and your glasses if you wear them.

Exercise one. Lean back, head pressing on the pillow, spine arched, tummy muscles pulled in. Hold the arch at a point just short of discomfort for up to ten seconds—start with less. Then relax. This is good for the spine and the neck.

Exercise two. Sit up, slide your hands down your legs as far as they will comfortably go. Slightly, gently, bend the elbows outward and hold this position, just short of discomfort, for up to ten seconds. Relax. Repeat once. Also for spine, convex instead of concave.

Exercise three. Lean back on the pillow again, feet still extended. If they reach the end of the bath tub, press each foot alternately against the bath. If they don't reach, stretch each leg as far as it will go first with the toes pointed, then with the heels pointed. Hold each position up to ten seconds. Good for the knees and hip joints.

Exercise four. Sit up, spine straight, arms stretched out in front of you, parallel and with fists clenched. Push fists out alternately, hold extended position five seconds. Three times each fist. Good for shoulder girdle, neck and elbows.

Exercise five. Relax back on to pillow, breathe in through the nose, out through the mouth. Hold each breath a few seconds. This may not help your arthritis, but it is very good for *you.*

Exercise six. Lean back on pillow, feet stretched out in front. Circle each foot clockwise, then counterclockwise, four circles each way, each foot. Then play the piano with your toes. Good for ankle and toe joints.

Exercise seven. Sit up straight, bend your head forward, backward, sideways to the left, sideways to the right, look over the left shoulder, look over the right shoulder. Hold each position five seconds. Then slowly circle the head on the neck clockwise then counterclockwise. Good for the shoulder girdle, top of spine and neck.

Exercise eight. Lean back on pillow, pull left knee to chest clasping it as close to the chest as possible, stretching the right leg out in front and slightly arching spine. Hold five seconds then reverse legs.

Exercise nine. Repeat number five but instead of lying back bring the head forward so that the forehead is as close to the knee as possible. Good for the back of the neck and top of spine giving them the reverse action to number eight.

Exercise ten. Stretch your arms out in front of you, shoulder level. Circle the hands from the wrists clockwise and counterclockwise. Move and stretch the fingers or clasp and squeeze sponges or washcloths. Good for arms, wrists and fingers.

Do these exercises without strain but hold the ultimate position for a few seconds. Repetition is not as important as the hold. After a few weeks you will find each position becomes easier. Neither seawater nor exercise are likely to cure advanced arthritis, but they may help considerably to lessen the symptoms.

Eat Seaweed and Live to be 200

SOMETIMES WHEN you glance down on the sea from an airplane, you see large orange-brown areas that look almost like freckles. If the plane happens to go low enough, you can see that this is seaweed floating on the surface. At beach level some part of it is washed up with the tide.

Seaweed is not very beautiful, either on the sea or on the shore. It looks more attractive growing under water, waving gracefully from side to side with the movement of the currents. Seaweed, however, is valuable. It contains splendid minerals which, when the seaweed is used to fertilize the soil, enriches it vastly so that plants which grow on it and animals or people who feed from the plants get a first-rate supply of minerals and vitamins often lacking in the products from today's devitalized soils.

Ever since I can remember taking any interest in seaweed, and perhaps since the beginning of the human race, the value of sea plants has been recognized. Over seventeen hundred different species of algae, of which seaweed is the most familiar, have been classified. Primarily, they are divided into four categories: red, brown, green, and blue-green. W. A. P. Black, of the Institute of Seaweed Research, said in 1952: "From time immemorial man has utilized seaweeds for food. In the Chinese Book of Poetry written in the time of Confucius (between 800 and 600 BC) there is a poem that mentions a housewife who cooks seaweeds. At the time seaweed was considered a food of great delicacy and even a worthy sacrificial offering to the ancestors. Several kind of algae were used by the ancient Chinese as food, and the brown algae, *Laminaria sacharina*, is frequently mentioned. In the East, seaweeds still form an important constituent of food supplies and are not used merely as appetizers or stabilizers of confections as they are in the West. Seaweed is used in Japan to a far greater extent than in any other country and is still said to provide about twenty-five per cent of the daily diet. The brown seaweeds, for instance, are incorporated in the flour and are used in almost every household as noodles, toasted and served with rice and soup."

In a letter, E. Booth, of the same Institute, just after he had returned from an international symposium on seaweed held in September 1965, in Nova Scotia, told me: "The Japanese cultivate a green alga and use the brown algae in soups. They also cultivate some unicellular blue-green algae as a nutrient for growing a mould or bacterium which is used in the manufacture of a fermented milk product, yakult. Edible seaweeds are used in China and throughout the countries of eastern Asia."

"In the West, seaweeds have never really been accepted in our diet," wrote Mr. Black, "and have only been eaten in times of scarcity and where the standard of living has been low."

Nowadays, there are quite a lot of ordinary uses for algae that we don't even recognize. For instance, many ice cream makers use alginates as a basis for their product. Strangely enough they don't care to admit it. Personally, since I found this out, I have been using ice cream more happily—I had always assumed it was bad for me. It's used in toothpaste, too, and blancmange; for puddings it is much better for you than cornstarch so I don't know why they don't put the ingredients on the package. In Scotland wrack is burned and from the ash iodine, bromine and potash are extracted.

A friend of mine who lives near the Gower Peninsula in Wales picks a bright green seaweed called laverweed right off the beach. You can eat it raw, like a salad, with lemon juice. Cooked with a little vinegar it is similar in appearance to spinach but I like its oysterish taste much better. Some people make the laver into small cakes which they call laverbread. They coat it with oatmeal and fry it in vegetable oil and very delicious it is. The Japanese also use this particular seaweed but they call it Nori. It is formed into sheets about ten inches by eight. In one year 6,000,000,000 were sold.

An alga that grows on the west coast of the United States is made into synthetic "cream" for coffee. I use it all the time, bringing it back with me from the United States where I go twice a year. It tastes exactly like real cream but it has less than a quarter the number of calories —for slimmers—and is an unsaturated fat for those who watch their cholesterol level.

Most people in this country, the ones who are health-conscious, find it difficult to obtain seaweed in any other form than pills sold in health stores. These are valuable additions to a diet but they must be counted more as supplements than food since they have no bulk. Personally, though, I have been taking them for a good many years off and on.

A long time ago, when I was a very young member of the staff of the *Daily Express* I was sent to interview a man who told me that a relative of his had left him a bit of seacoast in the west of Ireland. He'd gone over to have a look at it and found that there was very little there except seaweed. However, he was an enterprising man and he set out to discover whether the stuff had any value. He asked around, did a bit of research on his own, and received a good deal of help from various friends.

One of these informed him that it had been supplied to animals in a certain zoo and also to some of the birds, and that a great improvement had been observed in their general condition; for example, their coats or feathers had become sleeker and finer. The zoo people attributed this to the fact that the seaweed contained iodine. This seemed possible although iodine, at that time, was mostly used as a disinfectant for cuts or wounds. Still, they thought, maybe it had some value taken internally.

Another friend who lived in Ceylon sent him a cutting from the *Ceylon Times*. This was an interview with a scientist who had just arrived in the country and who maintained that "people might live to be two hundred years old if they ate seaweed."

The scientist was Dr. E. H. Baker, a very young-looking seventy-five, who went on to say: "Seaweed has always played a part in the diet of primitive man and savages living near the sea. It was largely responsible, I believe, for their freedom from disease."

"Modern interest in seaweed as a food," continued the doctor, "originated some years ago when a prominent expert on livestock feeding observed, during a study on cattle-raising in Europe, that the healthiest animals were those raised in maritime countries where they subsisted on dried sea grasses. This was followed by experiments on California cattle which were fed on kelp, large beds of which exist along the Pacific coast. So successful were these tests that further experiments were made on human beings and it was found that seaweed was extremely helpful in eradicating certain deficiency diseases."

"Actual tests," Dr. Baker went on (and remember this was quite some time ago), "by methods of chemical analysis have proved that about thirty chemical elements are necessary for living matter. Every now and again we are told of another element, so, in course of time, we shall probably find that all the ninety-two elements we know are contained in seawater, are needed. They are all in solution in the ocean. The only plants which certainly contain all these elements are the sea algae—seaweed. Seaweed is often used as a fertilizer for the soil by farmers living near the sea coast. I would crtainly recommend the constant use of vegetables and fruits grown upon land which is thus fertilized."

By the time I interviewed the inheritor of the Irish seaweed beds and read his various stories, he had set up a factory for converting his seaweed into pills. I tried some out and, young as I was then, I felt better for them. So I wrote the story using evidence I have given here and giving the name of a store that stocked them. By mid-morning of the day the story came out every pill in the store, hundreds of thousands, were all sold out. Evidently people suspected that they were short of vital minerals.

Last year I made a rather leisurely tour through Europe by car. Every day I had breakfast in the hotel where I had spent the night and then set off for a local market to stock up with provisions for a picnic lunch. One morning, in a German village, I bought a dark-colored, luscious-looking loaf. It could have been whole wheat but I thought whole rye was more likely. When I inquired, in my self-taught (from phonograph records) German, I had to look up the answer in my dictionary. It was *Brot von Seegras*—yes, seaweed bread.

Later I made some inquiries about this. For one thing, it was delicious; for another, I had it around for several days and it remained as fresh as on the morning I bought it and, as I later learned, there was no chemical added to the flour to keep it from going stale. I discovered that, before World War II a German scientist, Heinrich Linau, had experimented with seaweed from the enormous, seemingly endless deposits in the North Sea. He was trying to make, and he succeeded in making, bread. He couldn't continue his research during the war, but afterwards he opened a bakery laboratory in a small mill. Here he continued his experiments in the manufacture of seaweed flour.

He found that seaweed contains a certain amount of carbohydrate, but it isn't the kind that raises blood sugar; therefore it is not harmful to diabetics and it is not fattening. It has some protein and a small amount of unsaturated fat. It also has twelve different vitamins including C, a little D and the more important of the B's. The mineral elements number as many as sixty, so far discovered—twice Dr. Baker's count. More, people liked his loaves—they didn't taste fishy or of the sea.

Now, in some countries, they are using seaweed flour to add to wheat flour instead of the chemical preservative that often spoils the taste or texture and is sometimes positively harmful.

The Japanese use algae flour, too, to make small flat cakes which children like—and which are good for them not only because of the nutrients in them but because seaweed stimulates the action of the intestines—the peristalsis—and with a calming rather than an irritating action. It is said to be equally good for constipation and diarrhea. One type of seaweed, agar agar, usually red, and which forms a smooth, slippery bulk in the intestines, is particularly used as a laxative. The Japanese tear it from the sea with long hooks. They boil it into a jelly which forms the basis of soups, custardy-type puddings and ice cream.

My son said to me: "Why do you want to write about something with such an unattractive name as seaweed? If you must, at least call it kelp or algae."

"Well," I answered, "a weed is only a plant whose virtues have not yet been discovered—Emerson said that—and in any case that isn't even true about seaweed. More and more of its virtues are being discovered daily."

"Such as?"

"Well, toothpaste; the minerals are particularly good for gums."

"It certainly isn't beautiful," he argued.

"My houseplants in London are, though, you have to admit."

"What's that got to do with it?"

"I feed them liquid seaweed," I said.

People usually think I have a green thumb. It is really this brown liquid. And when we are at the beach house we bring a bucketful of the fresh stuff every time we go swimming and dump it round the trees and flower beds. This is nothing new, of course. Seaweed—fresh or liquidized—has been used for years and is the best possible fertilizer.

Artificial fertilizers, which may contain large amounts of the more important ingredients, often ignore the trace elements altogether. Yet without these little catalysts minerals like iron cannot function and so they lie around in the soil unused. It is possible for plants to be iron deficient on soils with abnormally high iron content—as, for example, in some Somerset soils. And we've already seen what happens when soil has no cobalt and what happens to animals and people who live on soil that has been overused and underfed: they suffer from deficiencies of many sorts.

When seaweed is burned, all the minerals and trace minerals that we need for health are found in the ash. Not everyone can bring fresh seaweed from the beach to add to their compost heap or to their garden. If they can, it is especially useful because it also aerates the soil. But everyone can buy and use liquid seaweed.

Some little time ago I went to visit the Ribena factory to investigate the making of blackcurrant juice. I talked to some of the farmers who grew the currants. One had recently tried liquid seaweed fertilizer on his crop. The currants were larger, juicier, there were more on each plant, and they were miraculously free from pests. Further, when analyzed by the Ribena chemists, they proved to have a higher vitamin-mineral content than any of his former crops.

It is obvious that only those minerals which are in the soil can reach the plants that grow on it, the animals that feed from it, and the people who feed from them. But the converse may also be true. The trouble with some artificial chemical fertilizers is that they often saturate the soil with an excess of one chemical to the detriment of others. Chemical insect sprays may get rid of pests—and people! Mysterious intestinal sicknesses sweep through communities and are given the catchall name of influenza. The Duke of Edinburgh, one of the shrewdest and most pertinent speakers of the day when he is allowed to be, once said: "Miners use canaries to warn them of deadly gases. It might not be a bad idea if we took the same warning from the dead birds in our countryside."

With seaweed fertilizer you don't need an artificial pesticide: plants fed with it resist greenfly and other plant pests. The seaweed seems to provide a defense system against pestilence of all sorts.

Neither cows nor horses get foot-and-mouth disease when they eat seaweed-enriched grass (or seaweed itself, of course). Horses don't catch horse cough.

This goes for people, too. The Gaedhealtacht fishermen on the west coast of Ireland claim that carageen is good for coughs, if they get coughs, but that they rarely do since the carageen—sometimes known as Irish moss—helps them to resist catching cold in the first place.

Even the ancient Greeks knew that seaweed was a cure and preventive of goitre, though they probably did not know that it was the iodine in it which was the specific.

There's plenty of the stuff around, goodness knows, and many people are recognizing its value for a number of different purposes. Food for the exploding populations, for instance.

"The Atlantic Ocean," said a Danish chemist, "contains in algae alone the nutritive value of twenty thousand grain harvests." He added: "If a cheap way of obtaining and concentrating them and making them palatable is found the world food problem could be solved."

Another Dane said that he believed that algae would one day play an even greater part in man's nutrition than fish, as algae multiply at an incredible rate under favorable conditions. Some can reproduce themselves a thousand times every twenty-four hours.

An American algologist believes that an ocean area the size of Rhode Island could produce enough algae to feed all the people on our planet if properly cultivated. "Whereas a wheat field needs one year to bring forth a crop, algae can produce fifty crops in the same period. One acre of land normally produces ten tons of wheat. In the sea, from an area of the same size, up to fifty tons of algae could be harvested every year. A great part of a land plant's energy is used up in its struggle for existence while little is left for the production of nutritious matter. Algae, on the other hand, devote all their energy to the production of nutritious substances. Thus algae are almost a hundred percent usable as opposed to only five or ten percent of land plants."

"Five million acres," wrote another American professor, "could meet the entire protein needs of the United States, whereas three hundred million acres are now devoted to protein production in conventional agriculture. If no other way could be found to turn this into food palatable to people algae could be fed to farm animals to produce meat, eggs, milk and so on to help meet the world animal protein deficiency."

"Off the Norwegian coast," said a Scandinavian, "brown kelp is already being cultivated on a larger scale than anywhere else in the world. This particular offshore region is especially fertile because every spring melting snows wash certain minerals from the mountains into the sea. Additional nutritive substances are borne along by the Gulf Stream, thus creating a natural sea farm in the area. Under the watchful care of the official government authorities, the seaweed forests are harvested several times a year. Before the war Norway used to produce sixty-seven thousand tons of kelp meal annually."

All oceanologists agree that there are still more benefits from seaweed—and the sea itself—that have yet to be scientifically proved. They also say that this is no good reason for not making the fullest use of this vast and apparently endless supply of foods, drugs and other miracles.

At least three, and probably a great many more, new uses for seaweed have been found to fit in with today's needs. Just recently, for instance, two different sets of scientists, one investigating space travel in space ships, the others looking into ocean exploration in depth ships, have found that algae can convert carbon dioxide into oxygen.

Had they grown it in tanks of seawater on the old sailing ships it could have provided a food which would have done away with scurvy—and should the need arise it could do the same today. Well, actually, of course, a vitamin C tablet could keep scurvy at bay but there is something nutritionally sounder in a fresh growing food than in a synthetic tablet.

Following along on these lines scientists are discovering that biscuits or wafers made of seaweed could be a valuable addition to a rocket ship's larder. One tablespoon of algae, converted into a wafer, has as much nutritive value as an ounce of the best steak.

There is a good deal of interesting discussion going along in scientific circles as to just how far seaweed can convert harmful strontium, from fall-out, to the harmless variety. The argument is a little technical to follow but in effect it is based on the premise that edible seaweed is already so saturated with natural strontium that it is capable of resisting the fall-out kind. The seaweed turns natural strontium into a mineralized sugar or sucrate of strontium oxide which is easily digested and acts as a protective barrier against the fall-out kind. Eaten over a period of two months, natural strontium can replace fall-out strontium. In addition, while land-grown food may be contaminated by fall-out, seaweed is capable of forming its own antidote.

Since ice cream, custard and quick-setting sweets all have a basis of seaweed in the form of sodium alginate these can protect children from the dangerous fall-out material, strontium 90, says the Medical Research Council's Radiobiological Unit at Harwell. They have found that it lowers the amount of strontium, formed as the result of nuclear tests in the atmosphere, said Dr. George E. Harrison: the alginate seems to grip the strontium in a crab-like manner making it harmless.

Good news for the pigtail set anyway.

SEAWEED AND YOUR BEAUTY

Whether you eat it, bathe in it, or put it on your face, seaweed is a really splendid aid to beauty.

Minks' fur grew very rich and expensive when only one percent of seaweed was added to their feed at one mink farm. I don't say that if you add it to your own diet you will grow your own mink coat—but it will make your hair richer and glossier. Or thicker, as it does with the wool of sheep.

It is true that the faulty diet of your ancestors or the shape of their skulls may be the cause of you losing your hair early. But if you have a picture gallery of baldheaded grandfathers, it is all the more reason to try to compensate with an extra amount of the nutritional elements which hair needs for its healthy growth and maintenance.

Hair which breaks and nails which peel are both brittle for the same reason: they are not being sufficiently or accurately nourished from the bloodstream. Civilization is often to blame. Primitive people, or those who live in places where there is little prevalence of choice, remain healthy until the white man's grocery store moves in. Eskimos, far from trading stations, eat whole fish and its liver, bones, skin, blubber and keep their hair and teeth until the trading station moves in and they can get white sugar, white flour, sweetened drinks, depleted foodstuffs. Then they fall apart.

I've mentioned the Aran Islanders before. Years ago I went there with Robert Flaherty, the Irish-American filmmaker, who was looking for a location to make a follow-up for *Nanook of the North*. He was enchanted by the beauty and strength of the islanders who were living on fish they had caught, vegetables grown on soil that was little more than seaweed, too poor to buy packaged groceries, drinking milk from cows who wandered at will over the flats at low tide munching seaweed, and eggs from chickens who did much the same. The islanders had thick black hair and strong teeth into old age. So he made the film *Man of Aran*. The actors, who were all island people, were paid with good (or bad) Hollywood money. After that many of them ceased to live the simple, healthy life. Instinct, which had kept them healthy through generations of adversity, was not proof against prosperity. Probably the Irish who were healthy on the fine, mineral-rich diet which kept their hair so black and thick, their teeth so white and strong, are now as bald as film directors, as toothless as tycoons.

Doctors and fortunetellers can tell a lot about a person by the condition of his nails. Uric acid shows up in lengthwise ridges. An illness is indicated by a cross-wise ridge; if it half-way up the nail the illness was probably six months earlier. Weak peeling nails, are often helped by iodine whether swallowed in the form of seafood or a seaweed capsule, or painted on. For those who use nail preparations, such as polish remover, look for the writing on the label which announces that iodine, "kind to the nails" (it's true), has been added. Silicon, also in seaweed, is a constituent of hair, nails and skin.

SEAWEED AND YOUR BATH

Last year when my husband and I were staying at our beach house, we carried seaweed to our garden to be used as fertilizer. My husband, who is an orthopedic surgeon with a tendency to arthritis, also used it to massage his knees and hips. There were two kinds of seaweed washed up: one was reddish and feathery, the other dark brown and covered with those nice pods that are good for popping. Both were wet from the tide so that a good deal of the benefit came from the seawater, but of course seaweed itself derives its nourishment from the ocean and therefore contains all the sea's chemical elements. The seaweed also provided a certain amount of friction and he found it an excellent "massage glove."

Then one day he decided to take it up and, instead of feeding it to a tree, to use it himself in the bath. He reported that, in a bath of hot water it was very comforting. He also thought that it had made him sweat a good deal more than an ordinary hot bath.

So I tried it. I weighed myself before and after—and found that I weighed a pound lighter after fifteen minutes in the bath. The effect, therefore, was rather like a Turkish bath: it opened up the pores. But better than a Turkish bath it also supplied a replacement in the way of minerals, and a "massage glove" to use in the bath.

I went into it more thoroughly later. Seaweed in a hot bath, I learned, does increase sweating and thereby helps to eliminate toxic substances. Dr. E. F. St. John Lyburn, in an article on baths for health, describes this action as therapeutic sweating. He believes it to be useful in the prevention and treatment of blood, kidney and liver diseases, as well as relieving pain in rheumatic, arthritic, fibrositic and similar conditions. It increases cellular metabolim in all body cells.

It is the poisons which accumulate in the tissues and joints, the organs and glands that prematurely age people. "Wet heat," says Dr. Lyburn, "is an efficient way to clean the blood of poisons. The hotter the skin surface the greater the activity of the sweat glands in the excretion of urea, uric acid and also cholesterol, sugar poisons, antibiotics, drugs and the constituents of bile and urine which the sweat glands excrete in greater quantities in water than when the skin surface is allowed to evaporate in dry heat."

"The sweat glands can lower the cholesterol and the ethereal fats of blood—the causes of hardening of the blood vessels; they can relieve cardiovascular disease by increasing the oxygen content and decreasing the carbon dioxide content of the venous blood; they can remove sugar and acid products which accumulate in diabetes,—acidosis and the uric acid which causes gout."

Dr. Lyburn recommends that any treatment carried out by people under medical care should be taken under supervision. But most people who just want to get rid of ordinary poisons of everyday living can treat themselves to a seaweed bath without necessarily having to go down to the sea with buckets. Of course, if you have managed to collect some seaweed yourself you can dry it and keep it for a long time. When you want to use it steep it in boiling water for fifteen minutes and add the resulting brownish liquid to your tub. You can also buy bath seaweed in muslin sacks and this can be similarly treated.

One well-known beauty queen adds liquid seaweed fertilizer to her bath. She claims that she can sweat off pounds (mostly water, of course, but also all those toxic substances mentioned above). She also says she keeps on perspiring for some time after the bath so she wraps herself in a huge towel and lies down.

You don't have to use fertilizer, however—though it is, in fact, just liquidized seaweed and perfectly good for the purpose—because concentrated seaweed extract especially for baths can fairly easily be obtained. You add a teaspoonful to warm water. I also add a spoonful of pine essence—I like its smell and the color it turns the water.

There is also a seaweed bubble bath which has a slightly piney smell and turns the water the color of the sea on coral reefs. This is called Algemarin and it has all the good of the algae—seaweed—plus the luxury of the bubbles. Well, actually, bubbles are a little more than mere luxury. The bubbles or foam are an excellent insulating material. The heat of the water does not escape into the atmosphere but remains with the body; metabolism is stimulated, the oxygen intake increases and so does perspiration. If the foam is maintained you can stay in the water as long as half an hour without adding hot water—which means your skin is getting the full restorative treatment—on and in—your skin. Algemarin, like all seaweed, contains the sixty known elements of seawater plus those whose value has not yet been discovered.

The makers of liquid seaweed fertilizer also make, from seaweed, of course, a splendid soap, so that when you have soaked as long as you wish you can then lather all the remaining impurities off your skin surface.

By the way, for those who doubt that the minerals can penetrate—though most people believe that impurities come out even if they won't accept that this can be a two-way traffic—let me remind them that iodine is painted on cuts and is known to penetrate—and of course iodine, as you already know, is one of the most important of the sixty plus.

To finish up and reclose the pores, after you have stopped sweating, towel yourself dry, rubbing vigorously. You have got rid of accumulated poisons, replaced them with helpful minerals, stimulated your circulation so that it continues to work at full efficiency. After that you should feel marvelous.

SEAWEED CAN KEEP YOU YOUNGER LOOKING

I have heard some people say that they do not want to live to a great age. This is partly due to the present-day attitude to older people. In some civilizations age was respected. This is not so today. Old people are often treated as if they were half-witted—almost always as a nuisance. If they are rich, people are waiting to read their wills. If they are poor, they are an economic disaster—mainly because they have been forced to retire. There seems little point living to ninety or a hundred if you have to live for thirty years or so on a pension with dwindling buying power. So most people say no, they don't want to live to a great age. But they do want to be young for seventy or eighty years.

Growing older happens to everyone. Growing "old" should happen to nobody. We should all be able to stay in the prime of life until we finally fade away.

In order to retain youthfulness it is necessary to supply the body with materials suitable for its perfect repair. It will attempt to mend itself even without the right ingredients, using any old bric-a-brac it can find in the bloodstream. But this sort of reconstruction breaks down. Sometimes Paul is repaired by something borrowed from Peter. Calcium, for instance, can be withdrawn from teeth if there is not enough in the bloodstream to mend a broken bone.

As a child I spent a very happy year in South Carolina.

Many years later I returned with my husband to find it very little changed and many of my old friends still living there. Among these was a doctor named Bully Weston and another doctor, an orthopedic surgeon, Dr. A. T. Moore.

As a hobby and partly as an experiment A. T. kept a chicken farm. He was particularly interested in developing hard-shell eggs. It was his belief that if he could find a way to make his chickens lay really hard-shell eggs, he could use the same formula to aid in bone reconstruction. He had developed a hip operation which could be even more successful if he could ensure a perfect union of the bones and, if possible, regrowth of degenerated bone structure.

There is one gloomy school of thought which claims that bone structure once broken down by wear and tear and osteoarthritis can never be regrown. A. T. did not believe this. He had seen many old people whose bones were broken and successfully mended.

A. T., Bully and I were all interested in nutrition and the possible benefits for hens—and people—whether or not their bones were broken.

About that time Bully Weston had been consulted by some racehorse owners who were wintering their horses in South Carolina. Of course, Bully is a "people" doctor, not a "horse" doctor, but he had performed many experiments with animals: experiments with laboratory animals can often help make people healthier. He had, for instance, observed the fact that the life span of animals can be extended—or shortened—by what they are given to eat. They can be made feeble, gray-haired and even dead—or kept young, vigorous and alive—by variations in diet alone. Cataracts can be caused in animals by feeding them incorrectly.

Their bones can be made porous, their skin wrinkled. Because animals have such a very much shorter span of life than people, poor nutrition catches up with them quicker and good nutrition heals them faster. From a doctor's point of view it is also easier to convert an animal to a good diet than a person.

Bully told A. T. that he had looked over the horses' menu and had suggested adding kelp powder, principally for its iodine but also for trace minerals such as cobalt, a lack of which can cause swayback in animals.

The horses flourished, won all their races the following summer and seemed to become immune from an attack of horse cough which attacked horses that had not wintered in South Carolina and that had missed out on the kelp diet.

A. T. decided to try kelp powder on his hens. Powdered kelp was added to their food and he was surprised to find not only that the shell was harder but the yolk also was firmer. Indeed, the yolk was the great surprise—you really had to jab it quite hard with a sharp fork to break it at all —and you know how annoying it is when you are trying to make a soufflé and the yolk keeps breaking into the white?

Obviously the next step was to see what happened to patients with broken bones. He started feeding them kelp powder and, for good measure, added bone meal and cod live oil. The bone meal supplied calcium, the cod liver oil provided vitamin D needed for calcium's utilization, the kelp added all the other minerals and particularly iodine.

He was quite elated when he discovered that the healing time on these patients was reduced by twenty-five percent. But those patients with broken bones were mostly young, victims of car or riding accidents or of accidents on the football field. Would it work with older patients with osteoarthritis on whom he performed his world-famous hip operation? He was delighted to find that it did have the effect of shortening healing time and even on the re-formation of bone structure in many cases.

If this simple addition to the diet—and kelp powder can be added to human as well as animal feed—can make racehorses run faster, be more immune to disease, help hens lay better eggs and, as we saw earlier, keep cows and horses free from foot and mouth disease, cows from tuberculosis, it must certainly contribute to a generalized repair job on the human body and help create immunity from infection. It should help in keeping bones from becoming brittle in older age groups—the result, not of age, but of an age-long deficiency of the minerals they need to keep them strong.

If you are a hundred percent healthy now with red blood, strong teeth, all your hair; if you are slim, vital, often congratulated on being so young for your years, seaweed may not produce any new miracles. It will just help maintain those you already have.

SEAWEED AND YOUR HEALTH

All sorts of medical remedies from the sea have been found, some many centuries ago. They are forgotten and hundreds of years later are rediscovered. Two thousand years ago Greek doctors used red seaweed as a treatment of intestinal disorders. Seventeen hundred years later a physician living on the shores of the Mediterranean learned that this same type of seaweed, known as Corsican moss, disposes of intestinal worms. In many parts of the world there are still sufferers from parasitic worms, and if the remedy worked two thousand and again two hundred years ago, why not now?

An abstract from a particular form of seaweed has been found to deter stomach ulcers. And as we have already seen, it has a lethal effect on bacteria of the kind that cause strep throats, pneumonia and tuberculosis.

There is something in seaweed, probably iodine, that primitive people realized was good for future mothers. One tribe will not permit young people to marry until they have gone on a special diet. With Maoris, for instance, the future mother-in-law has been known to walk three hundred miles over mountains to the sea to collect and dry seaweed. They have learned through the centuries it contains an element necessary for conception and the maintenance of pregnancy. Although it is considered "old-fashioned folk medicine," some mothers-to-be in today's modern, Americanized Hawaii continue to add seaweed to their diets during pregnancy.

When cattle have disasters in reproduction, they are given certain food factors, usually those containing iodine and other minerals and vitamins found in seaweed.

Dr. Claude ZoBell of Scripps believes that there are as many antibiotics in the sea as on land and that eventually more and better antibiotics may be found there. It is known that people—or their germs—develop resistances to often-used antibiotics so new types must continually be tried out. "This," says Robert C. Cowan, a natural science fact finder, "is a challenging area for research that will have to be explored if men are ever to farm the sea and make use of its powerful healing and antibiotic potentialities in full."

A seaweed derivative is being used as a substitute for blood plasma in Japan. It consists of large molecules of protein which are mostly excreted after several hours.

Phillips' milk of magnesia has an algae base. So have certain creams that are good for burns. Carageen, made into puddings, is used by the Irish for peptic ulcer sufferers. In the Orient a similar seaweed has proved effective in arresting dysentery. In Japan they find algae useful in hay fever. Obviously it is used everywhere to prevent or cure goiter. The Norwegians use it for vitamin pills, adding those few that are not already present. The pills also, of course, contain the sea's sixty known mineral elements plus ingredient X. In this case X stands for those mineral elements not yet isolated but believed to exist in seawater.

The Sunshine in Oil

JUST WHEN the earth's fuel oil—petroleum, that is—seemed to be running out and, in addition, the powers were beginning to doubt the wisdom of releasing all the atomic waste necessary if locomotion were to be atomically powered, it turned out that there was lots of petroleum right in the ocean. Well, where else? Because most people believe that it originated from the decomposing bodies of a thousand billion zooplankton and other marine animals and even plants buried beneath the bed of ancient seas. If this is so, there must be a great deal more of the stuff where a great many more of the bodies were buried.

Petroleum, however, since it is not particularly good for health and positively harmful for beauty, is not really the subject of this book. It isn't edible. A certain type of petroleum, known as mineral oil, was once thought to be useful in chronic constipation since it passes through the system, oiling the works as it were, without being absorbed or digested. As it could not possibly add any calories, some bright person thought of using it in salad dressing instead of vegetable or animal oil. This turned out to be a great mistake and was probably the origin of the myth that slimming is dangerous to the health. Because mineral oil, in passing through the system, gathered up en route every oil-soluble vitamin that it came across and eased them straight out of the digestive tract before they had had time to be assimilated.

These, specifically, are vitamins A, D, and E. A is necessary to the skin and the eyes, D to the bones and teeth, E to reproduction and heart; and these are only their chief uses: they have many others. A lesser known oil-soluble vitamin is K, which helps in blood clotting.

Petroleum has its uses, but it is not essential to life. People lived for thousands of years before the combustion engine was invented. Oil of other sorts, however, *is* necessary, not only to life, but to health, beauty and happiness. You've probably heard the story of the Texas farmer whose crops and cattle were dying for lack of water. "Why don't you dig a well?" asked a visitor. "I do and nothing but oil comes up" moaned the farmer.

When you think this over, you will see that the humor of this story depends on the values of civilization. I mean it's funny—well, isn't it?—that people should think, in this day and age, that life could be more important than money.

Mothers in the welfare state take their tots to the clinic and come back with nothing more revolutionary than fish oil. Remembering the struggle that their mothers and grandmothers had in getting it down *them*, they have been known to pour the stuff down the drain. How many realize that they have thrown away the equivalent of a month in the south of France?

The Vikings used to toss off gallons of cod liver oil. Their physical stamina is still, to this day, a medical and historical legend. They terrorized the whole of Europe for centuries. Their racial hardihood prevented any outside army penetrating their country all that time.

But there was another group of robust and virile people

whose effectiveness in combat and national survival record equalled the Norsemen. The early inhabitants of the Arabian desert certainly were in no position to eat, or even catch, fish. So it seems as if they had to have something else other than fish liver oil to give them their fortitude. And indeed they had. This something was sunshine. Hundreds of years and chemical researchers later these turned out to be one and the same thing. Sunshine and cod liver oil are the two major sources of vitamin D, without which the body cannot make use of the minerals calcium and phosphorous from which bones are made.

OIL AND YOUR BONES

The story of the cod goes back a few million years, the saga of cod liver oil a few hundred. Not only the Vikings but others are known to have flourished on it. The Icelanders always took it as an aid to better health. In the eighteenth century the Newfoundlanders had quite an important export trade in the stuff. They also used the oil of whales.

It has been said that it was the fisherfolk of the Western Isles of Scotland who first discovered that cod liver oil was a cure for rickets. In those days they only thought of rickets as a softening of the bones in growing children's legs; they did not associate it with a lack of sunshine—or, alternatively, vitamin D in the diet. It wasn't until very much later that the connection between sunshine and vitamin D was discovered—long after the oil was regularly prescribed for rickets in the Manchester Infirmary. This was two hundred years ago and was probably the first time cod liver oil was prescribed in any hospital.

At first British doctors were pleased with the results and increasing numbers of them ordered it for their rickety child patients. Then, as often happens, something new came along and they forgot about it. But just as British doctors let it go, Continental physicians became enthusiastic about cod liver oil, and at the end of the last century a British doctor was reminded of it by one of his European colleagues.

He had heard that the London zoo was having trouble rearing some of its baby animals—lion and bear cubs particularly seemed to be developing softening of the bone.

"Perhaps this French stuff might help," he said to himself, and went along to the zoo to inquire into the diet of the baby animals. It was lean meat, he was told. He suggested adding crushed bone and milk for their calcium content: it had already been established at that time that bones needed that chemical. And of course there was phosphorous in the bone meal also whether he knew it or not. "And try this cod liver oil stuff that the French think is so good for bones," he finished off.

Since vitamin D is needed for the utilization of calcium and phophorous, and since cod liver oil is the richest, and indeed one of the few sources of it in foods, this proved an excellent formula. The pictures of the gambolling cubs were charming, and were used by the newspapers, so cod liver oil's antirachitic reputation got a new boost.

Later a more scientific approach was made into the cause and cure of rickets, but a violent argument broke out in the medical press. One school of thought championed cod liver oil, the other emphasized sunshine as the cure. We now know that both were right. But it was not until 1920 that the connection was discovered and it became known that it is ultraviolet rays of the sun which produce vitamin D on the skin—provided there is some oil on the skin in which it can develop.

People who work outdoors in a sunny climate always get enough vitamin D. Sunbathers, who really work at it, often don't. For one reason they are probably not in the sun for enough weeks a year. Secondly, they all too often bathe or shower the oil off their skin before the vitamin D from the sun's rays has had time to be absorbed. Even though bathers often coat their skin with a protective film of sun-tanning oil this, unless allowed to remain on the skin for several hours, is less effective as a medium for vitamin D than the natural oil of outdoor workers which often remains on them most of the day. Or longer.

I remember once hearing of a child's nurse—a snob, as Nannies used to be in those days—saying: 'Little Honourables don't get rickets.'

Oh yes they do, though, especially if they are kept too clean, the sunshine vitamin washed off their skin and no cod liver oil to replace it. There are fewer Nannies these days and fewer rickets: mothers either know more or wash their children less. But there has been a considerable upswing in the disease in England since West Indian children, deprived of their native sunshine and unaccustomed to cod liver oil, have come to live in its smoke-laden cities.

There was a moan of horror among the nurses in one London hospital when a small Jamaican girl, whose appetite they had not been able to tempt, asked for a cat food sandwich. Children, before their instinct has been deadened, often know what food their bodies require. Cat food is, after all, perfectly good oily fish and who ever heard of a cat, even though kept indoors year after year, getting rickets? Cats get their sunshine from their dinner.

After the national health plan came into operation and cod liver oil was given out on a wide scale, rickets were reduced to a hundred or very few more cases a year except among the West Indians. But when a shilling a bottle was placed on medications, rickets increased considerably.

Animals are often better fed than people: people have no market value. The sunshine requirements for cows, pigs, sheep and horses are carefully charted, any deficiency for optimum health noted, and the animals' diet supplemented with the sunshine vitamin.

In England we usually get sunshine for rather a short period each year. It reaches us, in smoke-filled cities and through cover-up clothes, inadequately. And although sunshine holiday tours are becoming increasingly popular, they rarely last more than a couple or three weeks. And, as we've observed, a lot of the good is washed off. Even if it were retained, it could hardly last for the fifty remaining weeks. We may get a bit more from summer weekends or from certain foods, but there are very few of these. Some foods are irradiated; some fat fishes contain some vitamin D. But it is only enough to make us almost healthy.

This state of near-health may not catch up with us until we are older. Brittle bones, almost invariably attributed to old age as if they were an inevitable symptom of it, are really the result of a lifetime of mineral, vitamin and often protein deficiency—calcium and phosphorous, which come largely in protein-rich dairy products, cannot, as you know, be absorbed by the body unless enough vitamin D is present. That is one reason why, in those countries where women were, or still are, kept in purdah (and if they come out of doors at all they are heavily veiled and completely sun-protected) they develop porous bones even earlier than in this country.

"Old people," you will hear it said, "just naturally have brittle bones." In fact, the condition of their bones has nothing whatsoever to do with their age though it does have a lot to do with the number of years they have lived. If that sounds like a contradiction I would like to add just this: to the number of years they have lived on an inadequate or faulty diet.

"Getting a bit long in the tooth, isn't she?" you will hear people describe some older woman. And indeed she may well be. Because before even the bones of the rest of the body begin to weaken those in the jaw relax their hold on the teeth. These then become loose, the gums recede and often become infected. Next step, false teeth—known in polite circles as dentures. Sometimes even these have to be remade every year or so because the bone structure of the mouth has further deteriorated.

Adequate calcium and the means of utilizing it—that is, by getting a good supply of vitamin D—helps prevent tooth decay, jawbone rotting and even pyorrhea. Even quite late in life cod liver oil will help—although it is certainly better to start earlier—preferably in childhood.

As to bones, when calcium is not distributed around the body, they may deteriorate to the point of no return. Carried to the ultimate stage, the disease is known as osteomalacia (literally "bad bones"). At this point the spine and other major bones crumble and break.

This is rather rare, fortunately; it doesn't usually go this far. But who wants bones even slightly brittle? It just isn't inevitable, whatever the medical cynics say.

OIL AND YOUR HEART

They have dickered on the fringes of admitting it for years, but now the American Heart Association has at last admitted that atherosclerosis—a hardening of the arteries which precedes strokes and heart attacks—can originate as a result of a diet too high in saturated fat. A statement made by the AHA said this:

"Populations with a low concentration of cholesterol and other fats in the blood have a lower incidence of heart disease than populations with a higher concentration."

Eating less saturated fat; substituting the intake of unsaturated fats; cutting down on overweight (which is usually caused by too much saturated fat, and sugar and starch likely to turn to fat deposits in the body if not worked off in energy) were all advocated by the AHA as a means of avoiding heart trouble.

Yet men, and less often women, are struck down in their prime, many of them who are not overweight at all—but who do, usually, turn out to have hardening of the arteries. Peter Sellers was fortunate in being able to get expert treatment. Adlai Stevenson died before help could arrive.

All of this, of course, is related to the cholesterol study. Cholesterol, which nobody except doctors had ever heard of ten years ago, is regarded by most people as the villain responsible for many heart troubles. It isn't. As a matter of fact, it is essential to life. Without it the body could not manufacture many vital organs. It is the raw material of bile salts. It has a valuable function in maintaining the health of the nerves of the brain and of the sex glands. The trouble only comes when, through the intake of too many processed foods, another fatty substance known as lecithin is omitted from the diet. Lecithin is found to accompany cholesterol in natural foodstuffs, and its function is to break cholesterol into very small particles so that it can pass along the bloodsteam without coating the walls of the arteries. When manufacturers hydrogenate fats and oils they change the oil from an unsaturated fat to a saturated one and they discard lecithin. It is at this point that the hardening of the arteries really starts. As he cholesterol settles and hardens, the blood is slowed and heart trouble may be on its sinister way.

If you are interested in the technical difference between saturated and unsaturated fat here it is. If you are not, skip it—the explanation *and* solid animal fat. Accept it on trust that you should take your fat—and some is essential as we've said—in the liquid form of vegetable or fish oils or from the fat of fish rather than of meat.

For those who like to know the answers as well as the questions, here they are.

At room temperature fats are solid, almost solid or liquid. They are composed of fatty acids combined with glycerol, their character being dependent on the number or variety of those fatty acids present.

Three of these are necessary for life itself; they are called the essential fatty acids—EFA for short. The other fifteen or so can be used as fuel to give energy or to build various parts of the body. The three that are essential are called linoleic, linolenic and arachidonic. They are not obtainable except from the fat we eat. The body can make all the others from sugar.

A fatty acid is said to be "saturated" if all its chemical links are fully loaded with hydrogen. Processing oils—hydrogenating them—means that by beating them up hydrogen is added, lecithin removed. They lose their liquid quality and become solid.

Essential fatty acids are unsaturated—that is, some of their chemical links are empty. Some of the other fatty acids are also unsaturated. Oleic acid, the principal ingredient in olive oil, has one empty link. Linoleic acid, found in most other vegetable oils, has two empty links. The only oils that have several empty links, which make them polyunsaturated, are fish oils, the oils from fat fish or the oils from fish liver, especially of the cod.

Where there is a high incidence of heart disease in a population—the United States, Australia, New Zealand and England are among the worst—there is usually to be found a high level of saturated fats: animal fats, such as pork, bacon, butter, lard, suet, beef and lamb fat, and processed vegetable oils.

It has definitely been established that those people whose arteries are coated with an excess of cholesterol improperly metabolized develop coronary diseases more often than those who have only the right amount of cholesterol for the purposes for which it should be used. If it is not metabolized—that is broken up and distributed in small particles into the bloodstream which can then carry it round to the right ports of call—it can, as we said, cling in lumps to the walls of the blood vessels and stop the blood from flowing freely. Arterial traffic, whether in the veins or on the roads, is seriously slowed down by bottlenecks. You know yourself what happens when a six-lane road suddenly becomes only two lanes: chaos. The traffic can back up for miles. The same applies to the body.

An article by an officer of the Division of Industrial Research in Washington wrote that the oil from fish was gaining recognition as "a useful ally of both the doctor and the dietician in their joint efforts to prevent coronary disease."

He explained it like this: fatty fishes, and the oils extracted from their livers, have been shown by studies on both people and animals to be effective in lowering the level of cholesterol in the blood. These oils always remain polyunsaturated because they are never hydrogenated, the lecithin is never removed, the unfilled chains of the essential fatty acids remain intact and thus their health-building value is not destroyed. Further, they have a strong affinity for the cholesterol radical and therefore enable it to be broken up into smaller particles and distributed around the body.

If you eat natural vegetable oils instead of animal fat, if you have plenty of the fat fishes each week (herring, mackerel, salmon, sardines, pilchards are the most common) you will be helping to keep your heart healthy. But don't overdo the oil; it is concentrated and calorie-laden. While unsaturated fat helps in a reducing program in one way—it tends to carry excess water out of the system—it can add to overweight which in itself causes heart strain. This of course is especially so if it is accompanied by a starch food as it so often is. One heart specialist wrote: "Many factors other than diet play a role in coronary disease, including emotion and behavior patterns, lack of physical exercise, excessive smoking, heredity and too many non-fat nutrients." Or a lack of others. Even a magnesium deficiency may be a factor, he suggests.

Magnesium is one of the minerals that goes down the drain with the vegetable water. It is one of the minerals always in seawater and in the products thereof. This may be one reason why fish oil, especially fish liver oil, is better for the heart than many other types of fat. As it is concentrated, you don't take in many calories with it so it doesn't cause overweight. It contains all the minerals from the sea—iodine especially but also magnesium. It is polyunsaturated. If you don't like the taste, take it in capsules. You will get your fat-soluble vitamins, A, D, E and K in their own medium, along with the EFA and lecithin.

OIL AND OSTEOARTHRITIS

There is a certain oil to be found in a certain shell which may one day be of enormous value to the sufferers of OA. This is a slimy sort of oil to be found in a conch shell. It is chemically similar to the lubricating substance in human joints.

One factor in the complicated pattern of OA is that this lubricating oil tends to dry up later in life. Researchers are at the present time investigating the possibility of replacing the natural substance with that from the conch oil. Dr. Saul Roseman of the Rackham Arthritic Research Centre is trying it out in experimental work and later may find a way of using it clinically.

Thousands of books have been written about OA, and most of them agree that whatever it is *not,* and whatever it is or is not caused by, the result is basically a loss of smoothness in a joint brought about by wear. Some people are born with a tendency. That is, they may have inherited shallow hip sockets not sufficiently oiled by nature. Later some undue strain may set up a friction. Then there is a breakdown as there is in a motor car which has been overused and undergreased. So that if a way could be found to use the oil from the conch shell satisfactorily, and if it were used before the damage became irreversible, it could be very valuable. The warning signs of OA are there, long before pain or X-ray reveal them.

If you can no longer cross your knees as you used to, if your joints tend to crackle or snap with sudden movements, if your knees hurt just a very little going downstairs, if your back feels as if you'd been stabbed in it when you pick something up or you can't look over your shoulder when you wake up in the morning you may be running out of grease in your engine.

Except for the conch shell oil, there haven't been many suggestions from OA specialists as to what could be used as a replacement. Some nutrition experts, though, offer alternatives. They say, and, of course, they can prove it, that the right diet in youth is important. But no young person ever imagines that he, too, will one day be old enough to suffer from a degenerative disease. Some eat healthily and some don't, so that gets us nowhere.

Nutrition experts say: if bones crumble and break up, if there are deposits of calcium in places where there shouldn't be, this must surely point to a defect in the assimilation of calcium. Maybe, then, these bones were not getting enough vitamin D. OA is a joint disease and joints are bones and everyone knows what happens to children when they don't get enough vitamin D: they develop the deficiency disease known as rickets which we have already discussed. Calcium itself must, of course, also be supplied.

For rickets they are given cod liver oil. Probably the oil, if taken by OA sufferers, can't get to the joints, although some people think it can. But it can and does provide vitamin D which can and does help bone formation, and there is something else as well. Recent research has shown a connection between OA and a high concentration of cholesterol in the blood. Some—but only some—sufferers from the disease show sufficiently raised serum cholesterol levels for the relationship to be suspected. Maybe, then, it would help these people somewhat if these levels were lowered. It is generally accepted that unsaturated fats are effective in lowering blood cholesterol levels. Cod liver oil is more unsaturated than even the best of the vegetable oils. So that it would seem to serve a double purpose.

OTHER HEALTH BENEFITS

Scoffers and unbelievers will always tell you that if you don't get a cold, rickets, osteoarthritis, tuberculosis, and are not attacked by streptococci, staphylococci or penumococci, this has nothing whatsoever to do with the fact that you have been swallowing your capsule of cod liver oil. You might not have got any of these things anyway. And it would be pretty bad luck if you got all of them under any circumstances.

Well, we will just have to ignore that one and point out that the use of cod liver oil for tuberculosis was first reported in 1650. Its tuberculostatic properties and its mineral salts (for instance it has a higher iodine content than any other food) were reported in the medical press of 1909, 1919, and 1938. In 1955 a California doctor named Getz reported cures in his sanitarium and attributed these to the unsaponifiable matter in the oil—that is to say, to the mineral salts. Other doctors believe that the antitubercular properties are associated with the glycerol ethers present in the oil. The desperate mothers of small immigrant children, who are particularly prone to the disease, don't mind what's in it as long as cod liver oil cures the child.

And what is in it, exactly? Because vitamin D can be produced synthetically and there are other sources of unsaturated fat. But as with many other synthetic foodstuffs that vital ingredient X which nobody has yet isolated is missing in the vitamin reproduction, just as it is in a faithful, exact copy of a Gauguin or a Rembrandt. In a painting it is the spark of genius and in a food it is the spark of life.

For instance, in 1956, in an article in the *British Medical*

Journal, Dr. E. Watson Williams said that he had found natural cod liver oil helped prevent colds while synthetic D did not.

So what is it in cod liver oil that makes it lethal to some of the more unpleasant bacteria—the one that causes strep throat, for one, and the bug responsible for pneumonia? Then there is the staphylococcus—"stap," the hospital bug which can sweep through a hospital causing enormous harm and even death if it gets out of hand. It must be ingredient X, the essence of life, which man can't duplicate as yet.

Quite possibly shark oil also contains the unknown factor. Bermudians swear by a cough medicine which is one-third shark oil, one-third honey in the comb and one-third black rum. But black rum is powerful stuff and maybe, after a few doses, you would no longer be feeling any pain. Bermudians use shark oil as a barometer too, to tell them when a hurricane is looming. If you think that a hurricane has nothing to do with health you have never been in a Bermuda hurricane. It's quite an unhealthy experience. But it's true, I've seen it for myself, that when Bermuda weather is due to be fine the oil is translucent and golden. When hurricane weather is on its way the shark oil bubbles and boils, clouds over in a great turmoil, gets thick, soupy and angry looking. There just possibly is a scientific reason for this. The oil, dead or alive, acting as a barometer, may be influenced by various pressures. It could, after all, be useful to a shark to know when a storm is blowing up.

BEAUTY BENEFITS OF OIL

Since we are on the subject of shark oil you might like to know how sharks help to protect your beauty. Looks do count for a good deal. For instance, why do we hate a shark and love a dolphin, despise rats but are charmed by squirrels? It's just something about the way they look. I read the other day that young rats develop faster on a diet of shark liver oil than on any other substance but who wants young rats anyway?

But of course we do want young and healthy and beautiful, wrinkle-free skins. Here shark oil can do quite a bit. What you put on your skin may help a good deal but what you can get into it, under the top layer, is much more useful.

Of course, you must really start even lower down than the skin, with the muscles, the connective tissue, the bloodstream. A drop of blood can pass from a certain point in the body and get right round to base in six seconds flat, carrying with it food and oxygen to all the tissues of the body. First-quality blood naturally carries first-quality materials. It is these materials from which your face was originally made and is largely maintained.

I have often heard doctors say that skin can't eat skin food. By this they mean that skin cannot absorb what is put on the outside. They are not consistent about this, though, since they prescribe salves for skin disorders, massage creams for rheumatism, lotions for sunburn and a variety of other panacea for a variety of other conditions.

As a matter of fact it has always been known by the medical profession that some substances, placed on the skin, are quickly absorbed into the bloodstream and can be detected after a certain lapse of time, in the urine or on the breath. There is a massage cream used for arthritis (it is called DMSO) which can be smelled on the breath minutes after it has been applied to the skin.

Writing in the *Journal of Investigative Dermatology,* a skin specialist said that he had found that a component of polyunsaturated oil (which was probably fish oil as no vegetable oils are truly polyunsaturated) penetrates the skin within ten minutes. Another report said: "Materials injected into the epidermis, or outer skin, have been found in the general circulation. Materials massaged on the outside or placed on a plaster against the skin have been detected within the body. The canal system between the cells is held responsible for this."

Convinced? Well, anyway, the French cosmetologist Jean D'Albret-Orlane is, and so is his head chemist, M. Desperrois.

The House of Orlane specializes in products designed to help women who want to keep their skins looking twenty years old. Which is, of course, every woman over twenty-nine. To this end they have successfully tried out many living substances and embryonic materials. They use orchid pollen, embryo chickens (which could solve the which-came-first riddle); they have used that magic jelly from the bee which keeps the queen bee younger, more beautiful, more fertile than all the other bees; vitamins, serums, placenta are the sort of things that the House of Orlane uses to remove wrinkles, refresh tired skin and all those other marvels you read about in the beauty ads and always hope to accomplish.

M. Desperrois reasoned that while all these substances could perform their small miracles, bigger and better miracles could be achieved by getting them down to a deeper level where they could do the most good. A lack of elasticity, a dryness, a wrinkle, start under the skin, not on top of it.

It became a question, then, of finding a substance on which the biological products could be conveyed to the skin's basement. M. Desperrois lined up a number of promising conveyors such as lanolin and vaseline. And shark oil. He gave them each a different tint, applied them to the skin of a guinea pig, waited half an hour and then, with a tracer, observed what had happened to each of the oils.

The lanolin—which is made from the wool of sheep—and vaseline, which is petroleum jelly, had made very little downward progress. Of all the others, shark oil had reached the deepest level.

So naturally they decided to use it for a number of their different witches' brews. For instance, because it can go where it counts—where lines begin to form—the biological substance in Orlane's antiwrinkle cream not only rubs out (*atténue* is the word they use) existing lines—*les rides existantes*—but the substances also *retarde leur formation*.

The shark oil, therefore, acts more or less as a carrier. Other oils have their special skin-softening properties that they can transport without outside help. One of these is turtle oil.

Since we have already established that skin can indeed eat skin food it seems a reasonable assumption that when the natural skin oil has dried up—one cause of wrinkles as well as of dryness—an oil that most closely resembles the skin's own production will do the most good. This, say the experts, is one of turtle oil's most endearing characteristics. Another is that it carries into the skin the sea's exclusive mineral, iodine, a healer and a disinfectant in any medium. Turtle oil also is one of the very few substances—perhaps the only one—which is naturally both softening and astringent. For that reason alone it is used with great success in the area around the eyes—an area which tends both to wrinkles and puffiness. A turtle oil eye cream controls both of these miseries.

Turtles have been swimming around the sea for a hundred and eighty million years and have changed very little in all that time, say archeologists who have examined their fossilized remains.

A few million years later, but still quite a long time ago as we count history, the ladies at the Court of Queen Cleopatra discovered the value of the turtle oil. An anointment of the oil was regarded as the height of luxury. It was said to be able to give to all who used it the gift of timeless beauty.

You may remember Huxley's book, *After Many a Summer Dies the Swan*. It was observed that the carp lived for hundreds of years and therefore must have the secret of long life. Maybe anyone who ate a carp could live longer?

This really may be true about the turtle. His life span of a hundred and fifty years, his life history of a hundred and fifty million years plus must be due to *something*. Some experts put it down to a certain enzyme complex. Be that as it may, research has established that the turtle's oil, or certain unidentified substances in it, do have a rejuvenating, regenerating and cell-forming effect which may or may not make you live longer but quite positively can make you look younger longer. Here again this elusive substance X, the essence of life which man can't as yet recreate in a test tube, can put some of this vital principle into cells that are wearing out, losing elasticity, forming wrinkles. It can, in fact, hold back the dawn of age.

Cleopatra and her ladies were not the only ones to discover turtle oil as a beauty preparation. It was also considered an invaluable beauty aid in the harems of the Arabian kings and the Arabian knights. All the perfumes of Araby may well have been needed to scent the oil— it has a strong low-tide sort of smell which in these days are removed with deodorizers. After that any perfume that the cosmetician fancies can be added.

The Arabian kings, of course, had ships that sailed over such oceans as they had then discovered and these brought back turtles for much the purpose that we use them today: to eat, to use as decorative furnishing material, and to beautify their ladies. The hot climate of Arabia dried up skins very early if these were not kept well-oiled.

More recently, I was told of a tribe of Africans who lived high in the mountains where there was searing heat by day and bitter cold by night. Such extremes of climate can be ruinous to the skin if it is not kept well-oiled (as New Yorkers, with their below-zero winter outdoor temperatures and eighty-five degree central heating indoor contrast have found, spending millions of dollars a year for just this skin-moisturizing purpose. The Africans, however, both men and women, were discovered by explorers to have wonderfully soft and supple skins. Their secret was turtle oil. So valuable did they think it that periodic expeditions were made by members of the tribe to the seashore in order to trap turtles and bring back the oil.

Some years ago New Yorkers themselves went wild over a youth-giving cosmetic made of a mixture of turtle glands and oil. It had so great a success that a rival firm, watching their sales curve plummet, put out the rumor that the preparation would grow hair. Nobody wants to be a bearded lady so women stopped buying. Alas the rumor must have been untrue because for a while men with receding hairlines rubbed the stuff hopefully on their balding heads with no success at all.

"Unfortunately we lost out on both counts," the former managing director told me. "Women stopped buying just in case. Men didn't grow a single extra hair. If the story had been true there wouldn't have been enough turtles in the world to fill the demand. But I never believed it myself. After all, turtles themselves are as bald as Yul Brynner."

As we said, turtle oil closely resembles the product of the skin's own sebacious glands which young skins contain plentifully but which tends to dry up as we grow older. For that reason it has a natural affinity to human skin. It seems to dive right in, softening the underneath layer and easing out wrinkles. Its disinfectant minerals help remove impurities and pimples or blackheads. Its astringent quality tightens up sagging elasticity. In soap it lathers like crazy, does a thorough cleaning job and doesn't dry out the skin on any part of the body.

It's not easy to keep your skin the way you'd like it to be, especially if you live in a city with its grime and fumes, its central heating, smoke and weather hazards. We can only do our best with these ravages of civilization. In ancient times, they used turtle oil, not only Cleopatra but also the Queen of Sheba. And they had none of the complexion hazards of our time. It would, you may think, be nice to have lived in those days without all the dry rot of present-day living. But if we had, where would we be today?

YOUR SKIN AND VITAMIN A

Your skin is not just a useful wrapping paper. It has a life of its own as well as the life which depends on the health of the rest of you. It is an organ of your body just as much as your lungs, your heart, your liver, your glands. It can regulate your temperature as accurately as any thermostat. It can reflect emotions, age, fatigue, health, sickness, overindulgence, anger, fear by paling or reddening, blotching, showing blue shadows, spots. Liver troubles cast a yellow hue, high blood pressure shows up in blue veins in a red skin, anemia in a transparent paleness. Under- and over-weight have their effect in stretching or sagging, and kidney troubles can cause puffiness. Faulty glands may produce too much facial hair in women, too little in men.

The skin has its own little factory and can make oil and sweat. Like the kidneys, it throws off waste. Like the lungs, it breathes. It can grow hair and it acts as a guardian to other parts of the body by registering pain if they are injured.

There are layers of the skin similar to an onion. Under the top layer, which acts rather like a waterproof wrapping, there is another layer, the lining. Beneath that are fibrous, elastic tissues. There is also a small and necessary padding of fat to help prevent dryness and keep the skin smooth and firm. This fat also is a medium for the fat-soluble vitamin A, known as the skin vitamin. Although it is also of value to hair, nails, eyes, mucous membranes, all of these are, in themselves, related to the skin.

When you say that beauty is skin deep, don't forget just how deep that can be—right through to the bone, in fact.

That's why we can't just consider what we put on the

skin. We also have to consider what is underneath, the actual ingredients of the skin itself, which can come from nowhere but your food. As well, we have to think of the skin that isn't actually showing: the skin that lines throat, nose, and all other body cavities such as eyeballs, middle ear, urinary tract and so on.

Studies made on mucous membranes of both animals and people show that either, if deficient in vitamin A, accumulate dead cells on which bacteria can breed. The liver tissue of people after an accidental death not only is healthy but contains twenty times more vitamin A than that of people who have died from an infectious disease.

A lack of vitamin A causes skin cells to die and this, when it happens to your face, means a dry, flaky, rough texture, and unless the deficiency is corrected new sin growth will be abnormally slow.

Fish liver oils give the best available source of vitamin A—for one reason, they come ready packed, as it were, in the medium needed for their utilization—oil. Polar bears and pythons are said to have the richest store of the vitamin in their livers, but fortunately the much more prevalent halibut is nearly as good.

Although many doctors who are not nutrition specialists claim that we can get enough vitamin A from a normal diet, nutritionists have shown that, even from rich soil, seventy-five percent of people get no more than 2,000 units of vitamin A a day. The amount of the vitamin that is supposed to be in vegetables rarely is: poor soil, canning, freezing, cooking, taking mineral oil and many other factors prevent it reaching us, even when it was there in the first place. Another oil-soluble vitamin, E, may also be lacking, and this vitamin is necessary to prevent vitamin A being destroyed by the body. Dieters who give up all fats and oils, often find their skins becoming dry and tough. Even where vegetables contain an optimum amount—which is very rare anyway—conditions may not be right for its absorption; at the best the absorption rate from vegetables is only about twenty percent.

But there is one favorable factor: it isn't only the livers of cod and halibut that can store vitamin A; our own will too—as long as enough is absorbed in the first place and not destroyed. The addition of vitamin E doubles the beneficial effect of vitamin A, and this vitamin is present in cod liver oil, which also has a good share of A.

WHERE THE OIL COMES FROM

Well, of course cod liver oil comes from a cod, whale oil from a whale, shark and turtle oil from a shark and a turtle respectively. Petroleum gushes right out of the ocean if they sink a pump in the right place.

But where do cod fish—and for that matter, halibut, herring, mackerel, sardines and all the other big and little fish—get the oil in the first place? From the same source as the petrol: from smaller things living and growing in the sea. First there is plankton, millions of infinitesimal plants and animals, so small thousands fit in a teaspoon. These provide food for very small fish and some large ones. The whalebone whale eats nothing else. Plankton is rich with oil among many other nutritious things. The bigger fish eat the smaller fish and the biggest fish (excepting the whalebone whale) eat the bigger fish. This may sound rather sordid, but it wasn't I who invented this survival of the fittest but Nature. Or, if you like, God.

The English cod fishermen sail from such east coast ports as Hull and Grimsby. They fish as far away as Greenland, Labrador, and Spitzbergen. They go where the cod fish go, and the cod fish go where the smaller food fish go, and in the colder waters the plankton are thickest, huddling together, perhaps, to keep warm. These busy little trillions have absorbed sunshine and turned it into oil. The very small fish eat it, the cod opens his big mouth and eats them and then he stores up the oil against a fishless day, vitamin D from the sunshine along with it.

Cod fish trawlers are miniature factories. The fresh livers are extracted within minutes of the catch being made. The rest of the fish is kept frozen, later to be turned into fish fingers or frozen cod steaks or other delectable and nourishing tidbits. The livers, fifty percent of which are oil, are gently steamed in a special plant and the oil released. This is stored in tanks cooled by the northern waters.

Back in port the oil is delivered to a refinery and motor tankers for further processing. An awful lot of cod have to be caught to make all the cod liver oil that is needed. One firm alone processes a hundred million cod livers a year. The mathematics are simple: one liver, one cod. But in case you think we shall soon run out of cod, each female of the species lays as many as nine million eggs a year so there should be plenty even given the hazards that the eggs in the first place, and the baby fish in the second, have to face before they are mature enough to have stored up oil in their innards. Some people believe that only one out of every hundred eggs matures into a full-grown fish. But that still means that there are as many fish in the sea as ever came out of it.

In Norway's whaling center, Sande Fjord, the harpooned whales are brought in to shore on the whaling ships and these, too, are processed on board. The oil is taken for animal feed so we get it, like the cod gets the plankton, secondhand. We get it secondhand in still another way: some of the whale is made into fertilizer, on which grow vegetables, on which feed animals—which, again, we probably eat. Nature, with a little assistance from Man, fixed all that up, too.

Perhaps the reason we don't like sharks is that, from time to time they reverse the process. They eat man. If they can catch one. At other times they eat quite large fish. One day last summer I watched one of them at it.

Our family has an island in Bermuda on which we have a house. Nobody else lives on this island, which is situated in a lagoon to which there is only a rather narrow inlet from the ocean. From time to time, though, large fish come in with the tide and swim around: whip rays that look like Loch Ness monsters, amberfish and sometimes, though fortunately not often, sharks. Luckily these always seem to swim out again with the turn of the tide.

So last summer one of these got into the lagoon and for the whole day he circled the island scattering quite large fish—four or five pounders—ahead of him and every now and then grabbing one as it fell back into the water. Luckily, for fish and fishermen (not to speak of bathers), the now rather overstuffed shark managed to squeeze his way through the narrow opening into the ocean and that was all we saw of him.

At one time, also in Bermuda, turtles used to lay their eggs in the soft warm coral sand.

This business of egg-laying is so fraught with difficulty and often disaster for the turtle that it is really strange the species has lasted so long. Perhaps it was because in the first few million years there were no people to catch the turtles or eat their eggs.

The turtle mother-to-be finds a sandy beach over the tide level and with enormous effort, and always in the dead of night—presumably to avoid being observed—she digs a pit. Then she deposits up to two hundred eggs, which certainly allows for quite a few to be expendable. Then she carefully flips the sand back over the eggs. After all this effort she scuttles her weary way back to the water, leaving her offspring to lie in the hot sand until they hatch out and wriggle to the surface. Some people say that the hazardous scurry to the sea which they make at this point is less to avoid danger, or from an instinct for water, than because it is easier to go down hill. This seems to me a point impossible to prove. But down they go, watched eagerly by hungry sea birds on a lookout for this tasty, easy-to-catch delicacy.

Quite a few manage to get by the birds. When you add people, though, it's a bit much. The accidental arrival—they'd been shipwrecked—of the first colonizers of Bermuda ate not only the baby turtles but also the eggs and the mothers too, when they could catch them. Now, three hundred and fifty years later, they are trying to attract turtles back to Bermuda. Turtle soup is considered, there, as elsewhere, a great delicacy, though Bermuda turtle soup is entirely different from the kind you will get at lavish London banquets. This often is clear with small chunks of slimy meat (I have more to say about turtle soup and the recipe Caribbean-style later). Bermuda turtle soup is thick, rich, and those few Bermudians who know the recipe pass it in secret to their heirs on the day they are absolutely sure they are dying. By word of mouth.

The first settlers on these reef-protected islands not only ate the turtles and used their shells but they also discovered, while roasting the flesh over open fires, that the oil which the heat brought out cured sores that weeks of sailing and poor diet had caused. And because of the green turtle's commercial value to the cosmetic industry, the Bermudians have still another reason for hospitably inviting the turtle to return to their sandy beaches.

Most of the turtles nowadays are caught in the less well inhabited islands further to the south. One way, used by adventurous islanders (who, like trout fishermen, scorn the easy net) is to first catch a sucking fish, tie a line to its tail and then locate a turtle and throw the sucking fish at or near it. It attaches itself to the underside of the turtle and its suckers are so powerful that smaller turtles can be pulled in by the line. Bigger ones may have to have help from a diver to get them into a boat.

Native divers in the Torres Strait consider it great sport to ride a turtle. They are quite adept at steering up and down and sideways by pressure with their knees on the shell. They even have races.

The Sea Dwellers

THOSE WHO know about it say that the sea thundered against the barren rocks of the earth for a thousand million years before there was any stirring of life. That stirring took place in the waters of the ocean. Whether you believe, with the Hebrew and Christian religions, that God commanded: "Let the waters bring forth abundantly the moving creature that hath life," or with scientists of any or no religion who say they were chemically evolved, there is no disagreement that the first life did begin in the sea.

In fact, the first living things were not animals at all but plants. Having somehow evolved, these lived on the surface of the ocean, were warmed by the sun and developed a process by which they could use sunshine to make food from the dissolved chemicals in the water.

This process, which is still known only to plants, whether on land or in the sea, is called photosynthesis. Plants use a sort of miracle emerald-green substance called chlorophyll whereby oxygen is released and sugars and starches created. This is another of those processes which man, however brilliant at getting to the moon or devising total destruction, has not been able to duplicate.

Chlorophyll, this magic substance which can grab sunshine and use it for energy, is made up of carbon, nitrogen, and magnesium. The energy sets up a chain reaction whereby plants, on land or sea, release oxygen for us to breathe and create food on which we can live. It did the same for the first animal creatures—little one-celled beings not much different from plants.

Evolution has an ordered pattern which is hard to account for and I am not going into the metaphysics of it here. If we don't yet understand why things happen, we do know that happen they did. Eventually the infinitesimal plants and one-celled animals, free-floating on the oceans of the world, developed into higher species but there are uncounted trillions still around today and very valuable they are.

Somebody named them plankton. Maybe it was a Greek, or perhaps a Greek scholar. Anyway, the word comes from the Greek word meaning to wander. In other words plankton, whether plant or animal (phytoplankton or zooplankton), are not attached and have no means of locomotion. They drift where the tides of the world take them.

Plankton are important because all animal life in the ocean is dependent on them. They form the food of many small fish. Some of these fish, the diatoms, are so small that another only slightly larger fish, the copepods, can eat 120,000 of them in a day. A herring can make a hearty meal of 60,000 copepods every dinner time. The biggest fish of all, the baleen (whalebone) whale, lives and grows vast on a diet of plankton alone.

The tiny floaters contain protein and oil, vitamins and carbohydrate and minerals which make them a complete food. Professor Alister Hardy of Oxford, an authority on plankton, said. "It is no exaggeration that in plankton we may find an assemblage of animals more diverse and more comprehensive than is to be seen in any other realm of life."

Although planton have been wandering around the sea for millions of years they have only been recognized by man for a very short span of time, historically. Part of this knowledge has come from investigating their skeletons on dry land. In many places where the sea has retreated or where disturbances in the earth have thrown up mountains, the seletons of the little creatures have formed chalky cliffs—as, for instance, at Dover. Those famous cliffs are the headstone for so many sea organisms that there were half a million of them to a teaspoonful even when they were alive.

This sedimentary rock strata, as it is called, often contains valuable deposits of minerals, oils, chemicals. These can be reached more easily, whether for use or study, than those still remaining in the depths but they are just as surely products of the ocean. Substances such as potassium, gypsum, bromine, lithium and a great many other chemicals are all to be found in marine strata of this source. At a different level their oil is said to be the origin of petroleum.

Living, they can be of service also—increasingly as food. Indeed we have hardly begun on plankton as a food source. The sea can yield four thousand tons of food per square mile per year—of first quality, from the nutritional point of view and never spoiled by frosts, floods, or other weather hazards of the land. The land can produce, at best, six or seven hundred tons a year for a square mile, and far more manpower is needed to harvest it.

Much of the plankton harvest is converted into food for animals, but at least we get it secondhand, rather like the herring, and with most of its food value intact. In time it may also be more widely used for people—the Japanese make a very good fish paste from it, for instance, as well as soup cubes which are useful as a basis for chowder or *bouillabaisse;* they add both flavor and valuable nutrients.

Here is a vast potential food store for starving populations. To this end scientists are endeavoring to convert the flavor and texture of plankton so that it resembles the type of food to which people are accustomed: roast beef and Yorkshire pudding, hamburgers and sauerkraut, sukiyaki, curry, chop suey or whatever. Those who are hungry enough might be glad, even, of planktonburgers. Krill, for instance, the planktonic animal the Japanese use for their paste, taste exactly like shrimp.

But to go back to animal feeding. Some say that in time cows may need no land pastures but can be fed entirely from the sea, This would ensure meat, butter, cheese with a higher percentage of vitamins, minerals, oils and protein. Those pastures that still remain can be enriched with plankton fertilizer and can be used for growing other types of food.

To us on land—or, indeed, to those on the sea—the ocean's weather appears to vary considerably—from mirror flat to mountainous waves. But to the creatures of the water the climate seems more stable. The minerals and gases held in suspension and the aeration of surface waters seem to make the sea a splendid nursery for even the tiniest plant and animal in the thriving underwater community. Someone has counted and claims there are twelve million in an average square foot of sea water, but that doesn't quite seem to add up with the teaspoon measurement. Anyway, there are lots, and it is only in recent years, since the invention of nylon superfine mesh, that it has become possible to trap them in significant numbers.

Fishing depends on a profusion of plankton because where plankton are there fish go to find food. Certain types of plankton attract certain types of fish and experienced professional fishermen can find these even at night because they shed a phosphorescent glow.

One night last summer in Bermuda, at the dark of the moon, my son came in and said, urgently, "Do come out, the lagoon's all lit up." I gave him a quick look to see if it was he, rather than the lagoon, which was lit up but I put on my swim suit and went out anyway.

He walked into the bay and he *was* "lit up." As he pushed through the water he glowed: his limbs were illuminated with a nimbus of light. He tossed handfuls of quickly dissolving diamonds into the air, and at his feet small neon streaks darted this way and that, marking the passage of some small fish. I started into the water myself and the same thing happened to me. The night was dark and starless, there was no reflection of light anywhere. The water was lit up all right with the luminescent cells of trillions of infinitesimal living creatures. It was a very strange feeling.

Teeming millions are always important if only for their sheer weight of numbers. Plankton are important because on their survival and reproduction rests the entire pattern of the sea's economy. Since the people of the earth are increasingly looking to the sea for the food which will mean their own immutability, this is very vital indeed.

Life magazine once put it this way: "It is estimated that ten pounds of food are required to build one pound of the animal that eats it. Thus it would take ten thousand pounds of planktonic diatoms to make a thousand pounds of copepods to make a hundred pounds of herrings to make ten pounds of mackerel to make one pound of tuna to make one-tenth of a pound of man." Of course this pattern is endless, depending on the size and ability of the eventual trapper. A squid eats a herring and a bass eats a squid; possibly you eat the bass. But at the base of this pyramid is still the infinitesimal plankton, important because there are so many of them.

You could, of course, perform a similar sum relating to the land. This would, however, only prove how much cheaper food from the sea is than that from the land. The sea provides, free of charge, free of man hours, free of rental, all the initial stages that, on land, have to be performed by a landowner, a farmer, with additional expenses for seeds, fertilizer, machines of various sorts and of course water.

There is still the possibility that plankton itself will eventually become a greater part of man's food, but, like processing grass, so far it has been found easier to employ a middleman in the shape of a cow or a fish. Nature has had more experience in organizing these matters than man. But we're learning fast and in the future almost anything can happen.

In the strict sense of the word plankton—wanderers—all types of jellyfish should be included because they, too, wander without any personal means of locomotion. They are part of the chain of evolution, but so far they have not proved to be of much other value.

The fish that go most to market, as discovered by a British poll, are cod, haddock, flounder, and herring. That is what we buy most of and in that order. Furthermore, the poll revealed that from six to ten times more meat and poultry are eaten than fish. This is not only sad but also uneconomical. Fish is, in general, a good deal cheaper than meat and provides protein which is as good, or better, for fewer calories. You save pounds, and dollars too, if you eat fish several times a week.

The fat fishes—herring, mackerel, sardine, salmon, pilchards—or the oil of fishes or their livers—provide the only truly polyunsaturated fat in existence—which, as you may remember, is better for hearts. These fish also contain vitamin D, one of the few foods that do in its natural form, and also calcium. Neither of these is found in meat.

In the flesh, bones and skin of fish—and in small fish, like sardines, one eats the lot—are also all the minerals and vitamins that they get from eating from the rich soil of the sea. The bones, of course, have the most calcium. You also find these vitamins and minerals in tinned salmon. In the fat fish you get not only the unsaturated oil but also the oil-soluble vitamins—A, for example, and K. Many fish have B vitamins, too.

It's not surprising that people don't eat them, or not as often as they should. In England cod is usually boiled in water and served with a white paste sauce. Flounder is coated in a nutritionally unsound and not even pleasant-to-eat white flour batter and then fried, often in rancid fat. (Rancid fat removes vitamin E from the system which makes it very bad indeed for you.) Haddock, when smoked and served with a poached egg, can be quite delicious but unsmoked and boiled, with no herbs or flavorings, it is as dull as dish—or fish—water.

Of the luxury fishes—I judge by taste rather than price—a mackerel split and grilled is delicious; a grilled Dover sole is a luxury anywhere in the world you can get it; Scotch salmon, poached and served with a home-made mayonnaise sauce, is a gourmet dish. Skate, with black butter, is served as *raie au beurre* in the most expensive restaurants—and sometimes, fried, in fish and chip shops. It is rather rarely seen at the fish markets.

An old Scotswoman I know bemoans the fact that, due

to a shortage of oaks and oak sawdust, Scottish kippers are no longer smoked the way they used to be. I personally feel that what can ruin their fabulous flavour even more is the new trend for filleting them and putting the fillets in cellophane bags which you then cook in boiling water. This does, of course, make for lazy chewing, less washing up.

Fish is sometimes called brain food. Fish does contain iodine and potassium and phosphorous, without which the brain simply does not function. But unless anyone has previously suffered a deficiency of these minerals, feeding fish won't necessarily get them through their exams. But it won't stop them either.

The flesh of fish, like our own, is composed largely of protein. So, too, is the flesh of cattle, sheep, pigs, chickens and so on. But meat is more expensive and has a kind of fat which can be harmful, and most servings of meat have twice the calories of an equivalent serving of fish—which makes fish one of the best possible foods on a slimming diet. Fish can even be fried without losing its weight-controlling benefit, provided an unsaturated fat is used—corn, linseed, soya or safflower.

Protein is what we ourselves are largely made of. We need it daily to repair worn-out tissues—and tissues start wearing out from the moment we are born. Children, of course, need it in order to grow up at all. Protein consists of a number of ingredients called amino acids. These group together in a great number of permutations and combinations to make noses, legs, eyes, insides—the lot. Protein, from whatever source—dairy produce and meat, as well as fish—is broken down into its individual amino acids, and these are carried along by the bloodstream until they come to a place which needs their particular type for a special repair job—or for making new cells, organs, glands, blood and what have you. Obviously children need a great deal of these to make new growth. Old people, wearing out, need plenty for restorative processes. For either group, fish is a top-ranking food—it does all that is required of it and is very easy to digest.

Feeding in their rich marine pastures, fish can always get the maximum of vital food elements and pass them on to us. Land animals, in this respect, are as unreliable as the pastures on which they feed. These green pastures may be totally or partly depleted of the minerals that should be in their soil. Animals feeding from them will be similarly depleted, and so will people.

Why we eat from six to ten times more meat and poultry than we do fish is a mystery (when I say "we" I don't really mean me because with me it's about fifty-fifty. Perhaps I mean you?). It may be a habit. There is also some sort of strange tradition that fish is not really a proper main meal. At banquets, and in the old days, it was served as well as, not instead of, the meat course. At home it has become lunch, a snack, supper or even breakfast. It is rarely offered as the chief dish at a dinner party unless, perhaps, in the form of a whole salmon exquisitely dressed.

Some people think that Friday's fast accounts for this, even among non-fasters. They think that there is a psychological effect in the fact that fish is supposed to be a penance. I have often wondered just how this particular tradition or taboo started. It seems to me, as a fish lover, rather like giving children strawberries as a punishment. It must have come about, I fancy, through the great wisdom and insight into human nature of some early man of religion who knew how good for people fish is. Tell people to eat it for their health and they will be contrary and demand steak. But say that eating fish is a mortification and they will be delighted to find that their punishment is so delicious. Unfortunately, however, this piece of psychology has bounced the wrong way. Fish markets still sell more fish on Fridays than on any other day.

Although all the seas join up somewhere or other, the fish are not all the same everywhere. This is partly due to the degree of warmth or cold in various seas: the amount of sunshine and the heat of the currents determine this. Pompano, bonefish, swordfish, fresh tuna are good eating fish to be found in some parts of the world. In areas of the Atlantic there are grunts and groupers and rockfish, chub, scrappers and porgy, wahoos, yellowtail, and blackfin. Many of these are delicious eating. The Pacific offers still a different choice. Why can't we have them here? It is certainly not a question of refrigeration and transport. We get oranges from Spain, Israel, California, beef from the Argentine, butter from New Zealand, bacon from Denmark—you name it, they have it, we get it, so it can't have anything to do with the balance of trade, either. It is time we balanced trade with a bit of fish swapping. Scotch salmon and Dover sole are luxuries we could trade more universally. Oh yes, of course, we do get Canadian salmon. Scampi, by the way, don't usually come from Italy. They are Dublin Bay prawns, probably not even from Ireland, with a more fashionable name. Which just goes to show that now that people are traveling further afield each year, becoming more adventurous in eating the food of the country, they would probably welcome a bit of porgy. The name would sound excitingly like something by Gershwin. A promotion job is probably what is needed.

With seventy-one percent of the earth's surface covered with ocean it is not enough that only twelve percent of the protein eaten in the world comes from fish. And yet there is a tremendous world shortage of protein foods. Nobody knows this more acutely than the world fishing industry itself. They are all set to make aquaculture compete in a big way with agriculture over the next twenty years.

Of course, it is no good bringing fish to the market if you can't make people eat it. If they can get used to eating oysters, scampi and snails because it is smart, or if they are hungry enough, people will eat fish if they can get it. They can't always. I've been told of ships ploughing their way through dense shoals of tuna in the Red Sea, while Egyptians, only a short distance away, were either starving or suffering from that unpleasant protein-deficiency disease, kwashkior, because they did not have the know-how or the equipment to get this valuable food from the ocean.

Once upon a time men went out into the forests to hunt for their dinner. Then they started to breed, feed and market the animals themselves. With fishing we have scarcely reached the preliminary hunting stage. In the future, some suggest, fish will have to be bred and reared like cattle. Research is being carried out so that the farming of the sea will be scientifically handled just as farming of the land is now—with, we hope, more intelligence.

Without help from man, the sea can produce two million tons of additional fish each year. We harvest less than a quarter of this. Freezing, transport, canning and other methods of distribution are already sufficiently developed so that the half of the world's population which today suffers from protein starvation can be adequately fed.

If the sea can be worked as the land is worked, and actually it would need a very great deal less effort in the way of cultivation and fertilization, it can be made even more productive than it is. Since foods from the sea are complete, nutritionally speaking, and since they reproduce themselves very rapidly, it is largely a matter of getting them ashore and to the market. The White Fish Authority in England has made a start and hopes for more government support from the Ministry of Agriculture, Fisheries and Food. Certainly it would seem more profitable to explore inner, rather than outer, space, the sea's bottom rather than the sky's top. At least one of America's space men seems to agree. Scott Carpenter has spent a considerable time down under.

The seafood fed to animals is usually known as fish meal. In the last few years the world production of fish meal has doubled. A good proportion of this expansion is due to those wicked anchovy hunters of Peru who are taking the food out of the guano birds' mouths and the revenue from their own government's coffers. Guano birds eat anchovies and the Peruvian government has, for centuries, balanced its budget by selling to a worldwide market the rich mineral fertizer the guano birds' droppings produce.

The countries that use the most fish meal are Great Britain, the United States, Japan and West Germany.

In Great Britain we eat fish meal secondhand—by way of the food animals and birds who have received it. Just lately we have been getting a little of it direct—and why not, indeed? Fish flour is a high-protein concentrate of first order from a nutritional standpoint. It can be made into delicious fish chowder, used in fish cakes and in sauces to go with fish—thereby doubling the food value at a minimum of caloric cost.

I see, however, that there is some talk of refining it. I do hope that this does not mean that they intend to treat it as they do sugar and flour: remove from it many of the ingredients that do the most good. The Association of Fish Meal Manufacturers, however, hold out a ray of hope. They agreed at a large international congress that fish meal —essentially dehydrated ground-up fish—would have excellent food value as "certain beneficial ingredients" would not have to be removed by processing. They stressed that the Freedom from Hunger campaign would be a suitable vehicle for ensuring that fish flour is introduced to populations in need of animal protein—and maybe some of the rest of us, who would like a low-calorie, high-protein-and-mineral-food additive, could have some, too. We could use it in the right sort of foods, as we now use wheat germ— to add food value of an important kind to an otherwise depleted food.

World production of fish meal stands today at two million tons a year. Seventy thousand tons come from Britain's white fish industry. It often contains even more calcium than fish itself since many of the mineral-rich fish bones are ground up with the rest of the fish.

It won't be enough, say experts, with populations exploding all over the place and having to kill each other off to survive, just to treat the sea as the buffalo treats the mesa: as a casual source of food which just happens to be there. Fish are lazy hunters because their food has always been so readily available. Most of the time they only have to open their mouth and let it float in. The tiny fish open their mouths and in go plankton. The bigger fish open their mouths and in go tiny fish. For man it isn't so easy. Fishing is still a rugged profession and fishing wars can be just that. A short time ago the Russians, who have developed a fishing submarine, invaded the Bering Straits where American fishermen were still locating the bed of the much sought after king crab. They swiped the lot. An international incident was only averted because the Bering Straits lie about halfway between the northernmost points of both countries and it was therefore hard to prove that anyone was poaching.

Fish populations can be predicted. I once went to Woods Hole, Massachusetts, on my way to the tip end of Cape Cod. There are fish investigatory services there which specialize in knowing all about the movement of fish. As well as the Marine Biology Station, there is also a Bureau of Commercial Fisheries which can forecast the abundance—or otherwise—of certain fish. They also advise on how these fish populations can be increased.

As one pop song said it: "Everyone's gone to the moon." It is still to be proved that the moon will be in any way useful in feeding the "huddled masses." We know that the sea can do it.

There are two quite different kinds of sea species known as shellfish: those that use their shells as houses and those whose shell is a sort of hard skin. I was going to say those who can propel themselves and those who can't but I believe even cockles and mussels, as long as they are alive, alive oh! can make sort of primitive movements from place to place.

As a child, when you first find a shell on the beach, you don't think of it as something that once lived, a skeleton, a memorial. It is a thing in itself, of beauty, wonder, the sound of the sea (when placed to your ear) or a rainbow tinted jewel.

Shells, in the mind and imagination of a child, have their own purpose. A razor shell is for King Neptune in case he should think of shaving his beard. The slipper shells are the glass shoes of the sea's Cinderellas. A limpet shell is a Chinese hat and a cowrie shell is mermaid money. When you are a little older the cowries are used for nursery gambling, though their value is not retrieved in the form of coin of the realm. Some say these actually were used as money once.

Then someone tells you that a little animal once lived inside who could, by some means, burrow into the sand.

"You see those rings," they said (in my case *they* were a series of housemaids who used to walk me out in the afternoons), "if you dig down you will find a cockle. Some people eat them off a pin."

A pin? That seemed extraordinary. One must not put pins in one's mouth. "May I have one?" I used to ask.

"Certainly not. They are only for common people."

Like kippers for tea. Therefore sure to be delicious.

By the time my children were of an equivalent age we lived far from Lancashire beaches, housemaids and other snobs, and we had kippers for tea whenever we wanted. But we happened to be in clam country, and kippers, not being forbidden, held less allure. My children took buckets and spades to the seashore as children do everywhere and looking for the little tell-tale marks on the sand (so like cockles) they dug up clams. Meanwhile I collected driftwood and made a fire. Then we had a clam-bake.

In the evening, for supper, we ate clam chowder, a fine, fishy soup for which I will presently give you a number of recipes—it, that is chowder, can be made with different fish and can even be something like bouillabaisse. But Cape Cod chowder is made of clams, onions and potatoes mostly and is a very satisfactory meal after a long day on the beach.

Shellfish—the ones that make shells their houses—feed

from plankton. They open their shells a little, take in sea water which is always full of plankton, shut their shells and then dribble the used sea water out through a crack. And to prove they do have some means of getting around when necessary, you can see, if you watch, that limpets, for instance, slide round their rock to seaward when the tide comes in and so get the benefit of a fresh supply of plankton. When the sea retreats they slide back to their original position and remain there clinging like, well, limpets, to their chosen rock waiting peacefully for the next turn of the tide.

In Hawaii, where, of course, the sea and its products have always been readily available, legend had it that the food cravings prevalent among pregnant women were easy to explain. Says Dr. Carlton Fredericks, an authority on nutrition with whom I once worked: "It was believed that the disposition, health and behavior of the unborn child were determined in the womb and could be predicted according to the mother's food fancies. If her craving was for pilii (a bivalve which clung to a rock) the child would be affectionate and inseparable from his loved ones. If the mother's taste was for manini, which hides in the recesses of coral rocks, he would be retiring. Modern Hawaiians, Americanized, do not subscribe to those theories, which is unfortunate. Like many superstitions regarding food as practised by primitive civilizations, there were often some very sound nutritional reasons behind them."

Mussels are often to be found clustering closely around limpets and are, on the whole, more vulnerable. Well, I mean, they taste better, so starfish eat them and so do whelks, and then they are quite delicious as *Moules Marinières*. But there appears to be an inexhaustible supply, even around England. There was an advertisement in a newspaper a while ago for a "mussel man." He was required to be an honors degree zoologist and he was offered £32 a week, a laboratory, a two-year contract and as many mussels as he liked for his research. The advertisers were power stations on the south coast which were being bothered by mussels clustering inside giant conduits and getting swept into the condensers. The zoologist presumably had to come up with some plan to persuade them not to do this.

In North Wales, where the food supply—plankton—is good, some of them fatten to bursting point from overeating and these, like all mussels, contain a rich supply of minerals.

In general, mussels are not picked one by one off rocks though this is the way I have achieved them myself. At first I tried them out as bait and then, proving a poor fisherwoman, decided to eat the bait myself in mussel pie (a recipe for which is at the end of this chapter). Commercially, mussels are dredged for, lifted into sifters which revolve, discarding the undersized ones. These reattach themselves to rocks and grow to maturity.

British mussels are true blue, mainly due to a law having been passed. Before being sold they must be thoroughly cleaned in boiling water and some sort of disinfectant. This doesn't affect the inside or remove any of the minerals because the hot water causes the mussels to clamp themselves tight shut. So they can be eaten just as they come.

Scallops are among the most delicious bivalves in England except, of course, oysters, and there is a marvellous shellfish I used to have in California called an abalone. Unlike the oyster, the abalone put his pearl coating on the outside and as they are quite large shells and have ready-made little holes all down one side, they are frequently used as lampshades. The flesh is plump, resilient and delicious.

In England oysters are served on the half shell, in dozens or half dozens, at rather expensive restaurants. In the United States they are far less exclusive. For instance, there is an oyster bar in one of New York's stations where commuters face their crowded journey home fortified by a nice hot oyster soup. In New Orleans there is a famous oyster dish made with spinach. All over the United States they devil them, make them into a ragout with tripe, serve them with macaroni, piecrust, rice, with bacon, green pepper, anchovy sauce, mushrooms. Some of these recipes are good, and tinned oysters can be used satisfactorily.

Anything you can say about fish for health and slimming—and you can say plenty—goes double for shellfish, whether they are bivalves or crustaceans. While fish contain only about half the calories of an equal portion of meat, shellfish provide more gourmet eating for fewer calories than almost any protein food available. One slice of beef—376 calories; one serving of white fish—102 calories; one medium lobster—75 calories; ten large prawns—75 calories; ten medium oysters—75 calories; a serving of crab—75 calories.

Lobsters are not grown-up prawns and nor are prawns father to the shrimp, but there is, of course, a sort of distant-cousin relationship. On the other hand, early investigators thought they had found three distinctly different species in the three stages of a crab's development. I don't suppose the first person who found a tadpole guessed it would grow up to be a frog either.

Most of the shrimps used for the delectable potted variety sold in Great Britain come from Morecambe Bay, the Solway Firth and The Wash. They have to be hand peeled. What a fearful job it must be peeling shrimps day after day, week after week. High-speed workers can peel as many as two hundred in an hour—about 80,000 in a week.

For all their small size shrimps are crammed with nutritional goodness. Low in calories, they are high in vitamins A and D, minerals, iodine, calcium, phosphorous and iron. In fact, they have three times as much iron as a serving of beef and beef does not offer A and D. Lobsters, too, are rich in sea minerals and also contain vitamin B1.

Prawns come chiefly from Norway, the South Atlantic or the Pacific areas. Perhaps the outsize ones do actually come from Dublin Bay or anyway Ireland. There are specially warm currents along the south coast of Ireland, bringing with them fish that are usually found much farther south—even turtles have been found alive on this coast, and I suppose you could, at a stretch, call them shellfish. Anyway, Dublin Bay prawn is a fine large species which has only recently, with more foreign travel, become really popular and now even the frozen fish people call them scampi.

Crab is high in vitamin A and the B's and is exceptionally well provided with the brain mineral, phosphorous. The brown meat is more nutritious than the white; it is, in fact, the roe. It has a good proportion of unsaturated fat in this part. The king crab is much sought after. The Japanese can it, and export it; it is sold in our shops.

In Bermuda it is forbidden to fish for Bermuda lobsters (a type of crayfish which is clawless) during the mating season. It is even forbidden to eat them during this season if you claim the fish came from your deep freeze. How do we know, the law enforcers imply, that you even have a deep freeze or that if you have the lobster has been in there since open season? Not a people who trust each other, the Bermudians, and after the ups and downs they have gone through in three hundred and fifty odd years it isn't surprising.

You should always take the same attitude toward your fish seller. He has to live, after all. It is easier to fob off something not quite at the peak of perfection to customers who order over the phone. Crustaceans should feel heavy for their size and of course they should be—lobsters, I mean—over nine inches from stem to stern. They should be free from incrustaceans on their shells. This shows they have been around too long. I once found a lobster beautifully trimmed with coral flowers and the coral insect is not a fast worker.

Probably the first creature to come out of the sea and experiment with life ashore must have looked something like a lobster or a crab.

Scientists give no complete explanation as to where life first came from. Theologians say that God did it in seven days. If so, each day must have been about a million years long, a thousand ages for each evening gone. However, it is generally accepted that long, long ago, before monkeys and much before people, there was life in the sea. Although the earth was there it was not, originally, complete with snakes and snails and puppy dogs' tails and certainly not with sugar and spice and all things nice.

But the sea had something, the first stirrings of life in its slimy depths—or perhaps more likely in its surface waters. In those days life was very little more than a complicated set of chemical reactions which took place in a water solution of mineral compounds, but the sun played its part and so, perhaps, did the electricity of lightning. Eventually some sort of animals evolved and when the first of these left home to try their luck ashore, they put on a hard coat and filled up their tanks with seawater. The seawater, setting itself up in a closed circulatory system, eventually became the first land animals' bloodstream. Just as the earth is seventy percent water, so are animals and humans. And seawater and the blood in our bodies contain the same minerals. The hard shell which protected the first living creatures on their original adventure to dry land moved inside with evolution and became a bony skeleton.

But whatever the explanation of how it all started there is still a mystery. Scientists have discovered the spark of life but they can't, as yet, reproduce it. In 1953 amino acids, the building blocks of protein from which all animal matter is made, were formed from certain chemicals treated electrically and that was a big step forward. This gave the scientists the building blocks but they still did not have the house—the elusive spark of life, without which it wouldn't stay together, evaded them.

Setting up conditions which were believed to be similar to those existing at the beginning of time, scientists have proceeded even further and have produced a substance that looks and behaves like bacteria and has some resemblance to one-celled algae.

Psychiatrists say that in man the death wish is becoming stronger than the life wish. Certainly far more trillions of money is being spent to discover the means for our total destruction than to learn the secret of how to create life. There are others, the theologians perhaps, who warn that maybe the two go together and that we would be better leaving the creation of life and the date for Doomsday to whom it belongs.

Fish for Your Health

"LOW IN cholesterol and high in protein and polyunsaturated fat, the fish is gaining recognition as a useful ally of both the doctor and the dietician in their joint efforts to prevent coronary disease," says an article by Charles Butler in *The Modern Hospital*.

Low in cost, too, he might have added—which is more than you can say for heart attacks; they cost the country millions a year. Low in calories also—and overweight is one major cause of heart trouble.

He continues: "Various studies on human beings and animals have shown that both the extracted fish oils and the oils in the flesh of fatty fishes effectively lower blood serum cholesterol."

The fat fishes are, as you know, herring, mackerel, tuna, sardines, salmon, pilchards, all of which, says the article, contain the type of oil which is a compact source of energy and which promotes absorption of food through the intestinal tract. "In addition to its digestibility, excellent texture, and unique flavor, fish provides more protein for the money than does any other main course [so he did add that] while keeping carbohydrate, sodium and total fat intake to a minimum. A serving of fat fish, such as salmon or mackerel, will supply about ten percent of the daily requirement of vitamin A and all of the vitamin D. An average serving of either fat or lean fish will supply about ten percent of the thiamin [B_1], 15 percent of riboflavin, and fifty percent of the niacin needed daily [other B vitamins]. Although many inorganic compounds are found in fish, sodium is not usually present in quantities exceeding the levels prescribed for a strict low sodium diet. In short, fish has been established as the protein of choice in formulating anti-cholesterol diets."

Heart disease so often attacks quite young people without any warning. "He hadn't the slightest notion that he had anything wrong with his heart," you will hear people say at the funeral.

Better safe than sorry, to quote a phrase. There are said to be about two hundred varieties of fish and shellfish currently available (I rather question this figure, but I read it in a reputable source) which are safe for use in diets suitable for heart patients, or potential heart patients—those whose doctors have warned them and put them on a low-sodium, low-saturated fat diet—provided the product has not had the sodium content increased during market preparation—such as finnan haddock, kippers, buckling, etc.

Fish and other seafood are the ideal nail and hair diet. Although protein can be obtained from many other sources, first-class protein in seafood is also combined with all the sea minerals, particularly iodine. Fish, especially shellfish, contain sulphur. If sulphur is lacking in our food, we cannot grow either hair or nails.

Dandruff is cured from inside out when even quite small amounts of unsaturated fatty acids are added to the diet. The fat fish—sardines, herrings, salmon, mackerel, pilchards, crabs—contain unsaturated fat. One of the essential fatty acids, linoleic acid, present in the oil of fishes' liver and of the fat fishes, is essential to life itself but is also very useful in improving the condition of hair and making it shiny and thick. Dry, brittle hair and nails can be made as

NUTRITIVE VALUES OF THE EDIBLE PART OF FISH

[Dots show that no basis could be found for imputing a value although there was some reason to believe that a measurable amount of the constituent might be present]

Food, approximate measure, and weight		Water	Food energy	Protein	Fat (total lipid)	Fatty acids			Carbohydrate	Calcium	Iron	Vitamin A value	Thiamine	Riboflavin	Niacin	Ascorbic acid
						Saturated (total)	Unsaturated Oleic	Unsaturated Linoleic								
	Grams	Percent	Calories	Grams	Grams	Grams	Grams	Grams	Grams	Milligrams	Milligrams	International units	Milligrams	Milligrams	Milligrams	Milligrams
FISH, SHELLFISH, RELATED PRODUCTS																
Haddock, fried	3 ounces	85	66	140	17	5	1	3	Trace	5	34	1.0	......	0.03	0.06	2.7	2
Mackerel:																	
Broiled, Atlantic	3 ounces	85	62	200	19	13	...	...	...	0	5	1.0	450	.13	.23	6.5	...
Canned, Pacific, solids and liquid	3 ounces	85	66	155	18	9	...	...	...	0	221	1.9	20	.02	.28	7.4	...
Ocean perch, breaded (egg and breadcrumbs), fried	3 ounces	85	59	195	16	11	...	...	...	6	28	1.1	......	.08	.09	1.5	...
Oysters, meat only: Raw, 13–19 medium selects	1 cup	240	85	160	20	4	...	...	...	8	226	13.2	740	.33	.43	6.0	...
Oyster stew, 1 part oysters to 3 parts milk by volume, 3–4 oysters	1 cup	230	84	200	11	12	...	...	...	11	269	3.3	640	.13	.41	1.6	...
Salmon, pink, canned	3 ounces	85	71	120	17	5	1	1	Trace	0	167	.7	60	.03	.16	6.8	...
Sardines, Atlantic, canned in oil, drained solids	3 ounces	85	62	175	20	9	...	...	...	0	372	2.5	190	.02	.17	4.6	...
Shad, baked	3 ounces	85	64	170	20	10	...	...	...	0	20	.5	20	.11	.22	7.3	...
Shrimp, canned, meat only	3 ounces	85	70	100	21	1	...	...	...	1	98	2.6	50	.01	.03	1.5	...
Swordfish, broiled with butter or margarine	3 ounces	85	65	150	24	5	...	...	...	0	23	1.1	1,730	.03	.04	9.3	...
Tuna, canned in oil, drained solids	3 ounces	85	61	170	24	7	...	...	...	0	7	1.6	70	.04	.10	10.1	...

luxuriant as a cat's by adding fish to your diet several times a week plus swallowing a cod liver oil capsule once a day.

Vitamins A, D and E, the oil-soluble vitamins which need fat in which to flourish (in your diet, not necessarily on you), are in these seafood oils. Vitamin A, known as the skin vitamin, is important to hair and nails which, after all, grow from the skin. In fact, it is well-known that a shortage of vitamin A makes the hair coarse and brittle.

A mild deficiency of vitamin A makes the skin so dry that one layer sloughs off. This plugs up the pores, preventing oil from reaching the surface and of course the texture of the skin becomes rough. Also, the clogged pores often cause pimples to develop. Dry skin loses elasticity and wrinkles easily.

Vitamin D's role in skin health is also of interest. When the skin is healthy and contains its own natural oil, sun on the skin helps formulate vitamin D. It is wise not to wash the oil off the skin for at least an hour after sunbathing, or the vitamin D goes with it.

In California I once ordered a fish on the menu which was called Monterey salmon. "Do you mean that this fish was caught in Monterey?" I asked, surprised. "No—*bought* in Monterey," they admitted.

So first catch your fish. Or else buy it.

In Flatts Village, Bermuda, there is a dock where fishing boats daily bring back their catch. Sometimes I sail over from our family island to buy fresh fish for supper—I never could put wriggling things on hooks, or take them off, for that matter. There are usually only two boats there, and if you buy from either one, they will gut and fillet your fish for you. This is quite hard to do without the right tools and messy as well—another reason for not catching your own.

The fillets, which are rather coarse, are best cooked in aluminum foil in the oven. Spread fresh herbs over them if you can get them (on the island parsley and fennel grow wild). Dried herbs will do, though. Add a good dab of butter—these are not fat fish; they are something like cod—and bake them for about twenty minutes.

The Bermuda fish that are best to eat are groupers, grounts, amberfish, bonefish, hamlets, hinds and rockfish. You won't get them in England, but many English fish can be cooked similarly. Bream you can get. In Bermuda it feeds from scallops, oysters and mussels which makes it a very nutritious fish indeed.

The flavors of these, and most fish, are improved by herbs, fresh, if possible, dried if not. The three herbs that are supposed to be particularly right with fish are parsley, fennel and dill.

Herbs add not only flavor but also health benefits. Dill is rich in minerals, is splendid for digestion and is therefore used with cucumber to make dill pickles—the cucumbers are presumed to be indigestible. Fish have their own minerals, but dill is an addition to them; fish is usually quite digestible but some kind of cooked—or recooked—shellfish get a benefit from the herb.

Fennel has almost the same qualities; is also good for the digestion and for flatulence. It is also said to reduce overweight, but this seems doubtful, especially in the quantities used in flavoring. But fish in itself is a low-calorie food; even the higher-calorie fat fishes contain the kind of fat which is not "fattening"; it is polyunsaturated. Another possibly reducing quality is that fennel satisfies hunger pangs. The seeds have a slightly aniseed flavor and are very good in a fish stew.

Parsley is rich in vitamins A and B and most of all, vitamin C. It also contains iron. Unfortunately it is usually used to decorate rather than to eat.

Most Bermuda fish and quite a few English ones can be dry if not kept moist while cooking. They can also be flavorless if the flavor is not enhanced with such things as mushrooms, onion, shallot, chives, the herbs already mentioned. Some fish need mayonnaise, others are improved with caper sauce, black butter (butter that has been cooked a little too long), a poached egg, crisp bacon, and, of course, cheese. Cheese adds to the protein and calcium value as well as to the flavor.

Even fishes with their own splendid flavor are often improved with some addition. Salmon needs mayonnaise, grilled sole is improved with melted butter, a few drops of lemon juice. When you get fillets of sole in a restaurant very much covered with a highly flavored sauce you are probably getting plaice, or flounder. In fact in one cook book two recipes for *Sole Meunière,* one for Fillets of Sole St Malo (made with oysters and Parmesan cheese), one for Fillets of Sole Marguery (made with lobster, shrimps and Parmesan cheese), still another, *Sole à la Bercy,* made with a Bercy—shallot—sauce, start the recipe with, among the ingredients: "Eight fillets of plaice." On the same page, between Marguery and Bercy, is another recipe also calling for eight fillets of plaice, but this one is more frankly titled: "Stuffed turbans of plaice." Sounds rather good, too. The fillets are coiled inside buttered cake tins and filled with a mixture made by cooking mushrooms and onion juice for one minute in butter, adding a little flour (I use powdered mushroom soup when the recipe contains mushrooms and calls for flour. You then need no seasoning). When the mixture has thickened, add half a cup of canned crab meat.

However, it is not really true that plaice has no flavor of its own and has to be disguised as sole. Aside from its delicate taste it also has an interesting texture. But these have to be enhanced and preserved, rather than smothered. One way to do this is to cook plaice *en papillottes.* The French use these paper bags quite often because they really do seal in the flavor. One doesn't see greased cooking paper about so much nowadays because foil is so easy to use. Use either; grease the inside with butter, lay one serving of filleted plaice without skin on each piece of paper or foil, top with a dab of butter, sliced onions and a sprig of fresh (or dried) rosemary, fold the bag over and turn all the edges in securely. If paper is used, brush it with oil. Bake in the oven for about twenty minutes and serve in its own container. No salt should be needed if salt butter has been used. Let people add their own fresh ground pepper from the mill on the table.

Fish cooked whole in their skins are improved by marinading first before grilling. Make slices across the fish on each side, soak for an hour or so, turning two or three times, in a mixture of oil, herbs, seasonings and a little wine. While grilling, baste the fish with the mixture in which it was marinaded. If the fish is cooked in a flat fireproof dish, sliced potatoes can be placed around and also basted with the marinade. Both must be turned halfway through—about fifteen minutes as the grill should not be at top heat.

One another Bermuda dish is the traditional cod fish breakfast. It comes from the old days when there were no refrigerators and fish was often salted down in order to keep it. But you can use fresh cod just as well.

Salt cod is usually sold boneless and skinless but it must

be soaked overnight. Next morning change the water and add small peeled potatoes. Cook until the potatoes are tender. Take one egg per person, hard boil and chop it, add to it a generous sauce of melted butter and serve it with the fish and potato. Bermudians always have a peeled, uncooked banana with this dish; they consider it an essential. Nowadays Bermudians usually eat it as a Sunday brunch at twelve or one o'clock, and I have done the same thing in London with great success.

Bermuda's traditional Good Friday dinner is also of dried cod. Soaked, boiled with potatoes and onions, wild fennel and wild parsley (all local products but easily reproduced elsewhere). Then covered in a light pastry crust and baked until the pastry is done.

Some fish are cheap to buy because they are not much in demand and some because the supply of them is plentiful. But take, for example, whiting. This can be very uninteresting but it need not be. I cut off the tail and head, take out the center bone—not difficult—and put these in a pan with herbs and water. A bay leaf or two, for instance. This makes a fish stock.

Put the pieces of fish in a well-greased fireproof dish, sprinkle with chopped parsely and dill (or shallot or fennel). Add French mustard generously to the stock and pour it over the fish. Dot with butter. Cook in the oven for twenty minutes, basting at least twice. Drain the liquid, reduce it by boiling briskly, pour it over the fish and brown under the grill, watching carefully so that it does not burn.

Another useful white fish recipe—hake, cod, whiting, plaice—is made with mussels and the fish must be filleted.

Put the fillets in a buttered fireproof dish. Warm a dozen mussels in a pan until they open—or use canned or bottled mussels. Place them on the fish and pour on their juice.

Add half a glass of dry white wine. Season with sea salt and fresh ground pepper and add the grated rind of half a lemon. If, when the fish is cooked, there is too much liquid, reduce it by boiling and add a tablespoonful of freshly chopped parsley before pouring it back over the fish.

Here is a typically Italian dish which can come in very useful if unexpected guests arrive since it can be made without additional shopping—provided you have a can of tuna and some spaghetti and a can of tomato paste in the house. Oh, and garlic. If not get them in today in case your husband brings someone home from the office at short notice.

Sauté the garlic in olive oil until golden and then throw it away—the garlic, not the oil, of course. Mix this with the tin of tomato paste. Chop the tuna finely and if you happen also to have a small can of anchovies do the same for them. Add to the tomato mixture, season if necessary (the Italians think ground black pepper essential), simmer for fifteen minutes. Cook the spaghetti as directed on the packet, drain and mix with the fish and sauce, dotting with butter and sprinkling with chopped parsley.

Mackerel is a cheap delicious fish which is rather rich—one reason, probably, why the recipes of several different countries suggest cooking it stuffed with tart gooseberries. It should be filleted but left whole, which you may have to do yourself. It must be split down the back, and the bone, head and tail removed—but not too far away as these, simmered, are useful as stock in which to simmer green gooseberries. Purée the gooseberries, add seasoning and, if necessary, a little sugar. Fill the mackerel with the mixture, fold it together, wrap it well up in foil and bake in a low oven.

Mackerel can be made into an expensive dish by cooking it with champagne, but a dry *vin ordinaire*—white, of course—will do as well. The mackerel in this case is made into ordinary fillets, laid in a shallow dish, seasoned and sprinkled with chopped herbs—dill, parsley, fennel or whatever. Gradually pour in enough wine to soak in and fill the dish completely. Cover and bring to a simmer in the oven, leave to cook for five minutes and to cool in the oven until cold. Refrigerate and, when ready to serve, turn out on to a bed of lettuce and serve with mayonnaise or hollandaise sauce.

Prepared mayonnaise in England is peculiarly nasty; in America it is delicious. If you live in England you will have to make your own. I put the whole egg and the oil (soya or safflower) in the blender. Here is a useful recipe:

Take any filleted fish, the more tasteless the better. Let's say whiting. Brown a finely sliced onion in oil, add seasoning, herbs, a little sugar and two tablespoonsful of tomato purée. Pack the filleted fish neatly into a fireproof dish, cover with the mixture and cook in a low oven. Before serving, sprinkle with cheese, top with streaky bacon strips. Put under the grill until these are crisp.

I don't now whether fish eggs exactly count as fish, but you couldn't get them from anything else. The red kind which you get in little jars add a really gourmet touch to consommé and both of these can be kept in the larder against an emergency. You simply heat the consommé as usual until it is just short of boiling, divide the fish eggs into the right number of consommé cups, pour on the soup, stir and serve.

Taromosalata is made with smoked cod roe which comes whole or in jars. You put it into the blender with three quarters of a cup of oil—preferably safflower or soya though Italians use olive, of course—the juice of a lemon, three quarters of a cup of soaked, drained, brown breadcrumbs. It makes a smooth mixture after a minute's blending and is excellent with green salad.

Childbirth practices among primitive peoples are sometimes based on superstition but the superstition itself often has a fine basic health concept behind it. One tribe, living far inland, feeds marriageable girls fish eggs so that they will have healthy babies. Special expeditions to the sea are made to ensure the future of the race. All very wise because the fish eggs contain minerals without which conception may be impeded, or childbirth difficult.

Herring is delicious any way it is cooked, though its bones are a bit of a problem. There used to be a time when the fish seller would give you soft roed fish if you wanted: nowadays you must take your chance. So take the roes out of your herring—hard, soft or both—mash them with a fork adding chopped shallots, parsley and tomato pureé. Season and fry gently in a little oil. Grill the herrings and serve with the mixture.

It was a brave man, someone once said, who first ate an oyster. Well, perhaps there was nothing else. It was just as brave to eat, say, a raw fish, or a clam or whatever. There is a legend that a man, walking along a beach, picked up an oyster, it snapped shut, he withdrew his fingers quickly, licked them and wow! delicious! I suppose you can get used to eating anything, even missionaries.

The Chinese have been eating oysters for centuries but there must have been many oyster eaters much further back in the mists of the primitive past. Chinese, then and probably now, dry oysters and string them on bamboo sticks. The Greeks are said to have baked oysters in their shells in charcoal—which causes the shells to open—and then seasoned them with lemon and butter. The more one knows about the ancient Greeks the more one would choose their period in history to go back to.

This, and other information about the oyster, I got from a Mr. James Beard. I don't know which came first, the chubby Mr. Beard or the equally nourished Mr. Philip Harben (and who in the world would believe in a *thin* cook?), but Mr. Beard was sent to visit me once by a fellow cook (she had done the cookery pages on *McCall's* in New York while I was then the child care editor). What to give him for lunch? I chose grilled Dover sole which, like some wines, does not really carry and is never the same in New York even when flown over the same day. Can't think why.

Anyway, James Beard also said that most races who had lived near the sea—the French, Portuguese, Spanish—he didn't mention Italian in spite of the Romans—had learned to appreciate oysters very early in their history. He thought the best oysters in the world probably came from England—Colchesters and Whitstables, though the English had been known to ruin the flavor by adding vinegar. The most gourmet, best-known and longest-lasting oyster dish is Oysters Rockefeller from New Orleans. Some oysters taste coppery and indeed contain copper—which is good for your health but not your palate. In Prince Edward Island there are oysters as big as the palm of your hand. I told him that the oysters we find in our shallow bay off our island in Bermuda don't taste as good as the mussels which cling to our rocks. He said he'd been brought up in the Pacific Northwest where Puget Sound oysters were as small as a fingernail, coppery, but good.

While people in England serve oysters on the half shell accompanied by thin brown bread and salt butter, James Beard prefers rye bread sandwiches with sweet butter. A really party way to serve them is to put the open oyster shells on a bed of crushed ice and a dab of fresh caviar and a squirt of lemon juice on each.

His mother, he said, gave her guests oyster patties at supper parties. The oysters were cooked in a little of their own juice. The cream sauce for them was made with liquor from the oysters, cream, two egg yolks and sherry added gradually to the usual blend of flour and butter.

He himself likes oyster stew. You can make it with milk, milk and cream, light cream or even heavy cream. Add the oyster liquid to whichever it is, bring to boiling point, add the oysters and bring again to the boiling point. Season, pour into bowls previously heated and buttered.

Here's just one other suggestion for oysters, American but not James Beard. You melt two tablespoonsful of butter with one of anchovy paste. Whisk six eggs with a dash of tabasco. Pour into hot anchovy butter and scramble. Just before the eggs set, toss in the chopped drained oysters and finish scrambling. Serve with croûtons of fried bread. This is one of those five-minute dishes for unexpected company which depends on your larder. If you haven't any oysters, shrimps or prawns will do. But you do need the anchovy paste for piquancy.

The Greeks make an interesting prawn dish out of things you are not too likely to have all at the same time in your larder. But you easily may. Otherwise, lay in a stock in advance of olive oil, lemons, black olives and capers. And a pound of shelled prawns. Add a cup of water to one of wine, add salt and pepper and bring to the boil. Put in the prawns and boil for three minutes. Remove prawns and continue boiling liquid until it is reduced to one quarter. Set aside and beat half a cup of olive oil and the juice of one lemon together, add the reduced fluid, the stoned and sliced olives and a few capers. Put the prawns on a dish and cover with the sauce.

Mrs. Kitty Zuill, of Bermuda, gave me this recipe for mussel pie:

Wash and mince one quart of mussels, add a cup of raw diced potatoes and one and a half cups of cold water. Boil the whole for about twenty minutes until the potatoes are cooked, then add a large onion, first sliced and fried with small chunks of salt pork until tender. Combine this with a teaspoonful of curry mixed with flour and a dash of brown sugar. Place all together in a baking dish and cover with baking powder biscuit crust and bake in a quick oven.

The more international way to cook mussels is to drain and strain their liquid, add white wine and thicken slightly with sea moss (carageen), which adds to the nutritional and taste value of the dish. Put the mussels into a deep soup bowl and pour the hot sauce over them. Whether or not you add the white wine and call it *Moules Marinières* or eat it teetotal and name it stewed mussels (stewed? Well, only in water) the dish is of exceptional food value and is not even fattening. It contains all the minerals your blood, glands, fingernails and hair need. The protein is as good as that of meat—first-class, that is—and the fat is a great deal better than any animal fat. In fact, calorie for calorie, mussels—and all other shellfish—provide more than any meat in the way of health-giving properties.

Any cold shellfish—shrimps, prawns, lobster, crab—any or all—are delicious in summer served with grapefruit on lettuce. They also complement avocado especially when a sauce of half mayonnaise, half tomato ketchup is used.

For non-weight watchers, here is a lobster cocktail which I saw being made in a Dutch restaurant. I wasn't looking over anyone's shoulder: they brought the ingredients to the table and did it before my very eyes. The lobster, already cut into small pieces, was in a silver bowl over crushed ice. The waiter made the sauce by stirring brandy into a very heavy cream until they were well blended. He then added some tomato ketchup and blended again. He put some of the lobster into glasses and poured the sauce over. It is a fabulous mixture but it does rather dull your appetite for the rest of the dinner, which, in Holland, is a pity.

Here's another exotic dish, Chinese in spirit if not in origin. It's called Sweet and Sour Prawns. Marinade half a pound of frozen prawns in half a wineglass of sherry. Sauté two onions and two sliced green peppers in rings until tender. Drain shrimps and add a quarter cup of the juice from the marinade and four tinned pineapple wedges. Cover and cook from three to five minutes. Blend in carefully a tablespoonful of cornflour, two teaspoonfuls of soya sauce, a half cup of wine vinegar, a half cup of brown sugar and stir until it thickens. Blend in the prawns, cook for thirty seconds. Cover and turn heat off. Leave two minutes covered before serving. Serve with boiled rice.

Potted shrimps, the kind with butter on the top, are delicious with scrambled eggs. Melt the shrimps first, then stir in the eggs, four eggs per six ounces of shrimp.

Scallops don't need much fussing over, they are best cooked in the simplest possible way—removed from shell, the black part taken off, cooked in a little water until tender, replaced in the clean shell, topped with a white sauce (or a sauce made with mushroom soup mix), sprinkled lightly with breadcrumbs (I use wheat germ for additional nourishment) and grated parmesan cheese and grilled until golden.

I suppose chowder is of American origin. The French call a similar dish *bouillabaisse* and the Germans *Fischsuppe*, the Russians *Selianka*. We English don't seem to have a national name for it at all and indeed not even a national recipe. I hope this is not because, as Beethoven once wrote, only the pure in heart can make a good soup. The New Englanders claim to have invented the dish though even these admit the origin of the word probably came from the French, *chaudière,* a large kettle. The fact is that anyone who digs around on the beach and gets a fine mess of clams (or cockles or whatever) or anyone who sets out a net and gets a mixed bag of fish, probably shoves the lot into a big pan with anything else that is handy—potatoes, onions, herbs, maybe—and thereby gets a nice hot nutritious supper at almost no cost (if he's grown his own potatoes).

Clam chowder, the Cape Cod kind, however, uses no other fish. They make it with, say, two dozen clams they have dug up or bought fresh. We can make it with canned clams, three-, ten-, and a half-ounce size. Whether steamed fresh or uncanned, save the liquid. Fry a few slices of bacon, remove and sauté a cup of chopped onion for five minutes, add clam liquid, seasoned, and three cups of peeled diced potatoes. Add water if the liquid is less than four cups, simmer until potato is tender, add clams, two cups of milk, two cups of light cream, two tablespoonsful of butter. Reheat but don't boil. Crumble or chop bacon small and sprinkle it on top.

Manhattan chowder is similar except that in New York they use more vegetables, fewer clams: diced celery, carrot, turnip, and cooked or canned tomatoes. It's also good.

Bouillabaisse, which originated in the seacoast areas of the Mediterranean, is a much more mixed-up dish. They use white fish, mussels, lobster or crayfish, small crabs, conger eel, octopus legs all or any. In England the white fish could be hake, cod, mullet, bream, whiting, mussels, cockles—again all or any. You can even add, toward the end, a can of crab or lobster. They use the white of leeks rather than onions, add a bouquet garni of herbs (mixed herbs in a muslin bag). They often use garlic, nearly always olive oil and invariably white wine. Otherwise it is made similarly to chowder.

The Russians, in their *Selianka,* add capers and gherkins. They use any white fish but they also add some thin slices of smoked salmon, cut up shrimp and fish stock or clam juice.

The German *Fischsuppe* is made by sautéing white fish and onion in butter, using stock from the heads, bones and tails, etc., gradually stirred in. They beat a couple of egg yolks with the juice of a lemon and gradually add the hot soup, beating all the time. Reheat to below boiling point.

The Italians in their *Cioppino* don't use potatoes or in fact any vegetables with the fish but cook a white fish, a crab or lobster, shrimps, clams, mussels and oysters, saving the liquid for a sauce in which they do use some vegetables and herbs. Onion and green pepper chopped and sautéd, in olive oil, with three cloves of garlic, mashed, a large can of tomatoes, red wine, tomato juice, fish stock and herbs—bay leaf, parsley and basil, chiefly. The sauce is poured over the fish and all heated well, to below boiling point.

Actually you can make a very good poor man's fish chowder with just fish heads alone using the rest of the fish for another meal. Brown an onion with a strip of bacon. Place the fish heads in the same pan and brown. Add salted water and boil until the fish comes from the bones. Take out fish heads, remove flesh and replace in the pan, adding diced potatoes, chopped or dried thyme, parsley or other herbs. Cook until potatoes are tender and just before serving add a chopped hard-boiled egg. Since this is a dish that originates in Barbados you can also, if you have it, add half a cup of Barbados rum.

When turtle soup is made in the Caribbean style, it doesn't much resemble the clear liquid of the Lord Mayors' banquets with its fragments of jellied meat (experts can tell which part of the turtle it came from and call it calipee or calipash accordingly). I imagine the Mayor's cooks probably get this from cans nowadays. In the Caribbean they get two or three pounds of turtle meat, put it in a four-quart saucepan and boil until tender. They then remove the skin and bones, chop up the meat and return to the stock. Then they add two cups of clear beef stock and boil for a further twenty minutes. At this point you could open up a can and get pretty much what they then have. But from now on it is very different. They brown two medium sized onions in a pan with salt pork or bacon, adding thyme and parsley, and a teaspoonful of whole cloves. They tie all of this into a cheesecloth bag and put it in the soup with two tablespoonfuls of cassava flour—I suppose cornflour might do—add a tablespoonful of allspice and a teaspoon of nutmeg. When all this has been well blended, add a thickening of butter and flour and a tablespoonful of Worcestershire sauce, salt and cayenne pepper, brandy, sherry and lemon juice to taste. Serve finally (says this Caribbean recipe—and about time) with slices of lime and hard-boiled egg.

I've had this soup twice. It is extremely rich, much more even than it sounds. As it is usually the start of a fairly large meal one is wise not to take too much. The first time I had it, it was preceded by oysters, followed by broiled lobster. When the pudding was put on the table I took one look and groggily followed two other guests out of the room. All three of us fell into a sort of a coma and did not wake up until after midnight. I never did find out whether our hosts were flattered or furious. They made no comment.

GRILLED COD STEAKS WITH ALMONDS AND MUSHROOMS

4 oz cod steaks, preferably from tail end
4 oz butter, melted
1 oz parmesan cheese

¼ lb almonds, blanched
¼ lb mushrooms, skinned
slices of tomato, or tomato "flowers"
parsley

Using half the butter, brush the cod steaks and sprinkle with cheese. Grill until tender and cooked. Meanwhile, sauté the almonds and mushrooms in the remaining butter. Place the fish in serving dish and surround the cod steaks with the almonds and mushrooms. Decorate the fish with tomato "flowers" and parsley. Serves 4.

FISH SALAD WITH CHIVE DRESSING

3 cod or haddock fillets
¼ pint milk
seasoning
juice of 1 lemon
lettuce, watercress

Dressing
¼ pint thick mayonnaise
2 tsp of chopped gherkins
2 tsp of chopped capers
4 tsp of chopped spring onion tops (or chives when in season)
3 tsp vinegar

Wash and prepare fish. Cut into portions and place fish into a shallow baking dish. Season well with pepper and salt and squeeze lemon juice over the fish. Add the milk to the fish and cover the baking dish with either a lid or aluminium foil. Bake in a moderate oven 350°F for 20 minutes. When cooked, remove the fish from the dish and leave to cool.

Make the dressing as follows—place the mayonnaise into a mixing bowl. Add vinegar and lemon juice and mix together well. Add the chopped gherkins, capers and spring onion tops to the dressing. Prepare salad stuff and arrange lettuce on a serving dish. Place the cold fish on the lettuce leaves and pour a little of the dressing over each piece of fish allowing some of the fish still to show. Serve the rest of the dressing separately. Serves 3.

HADDOCK OMELETTE

1 fillet smoked haddock	pepper and salt
butter	4–6 egg omelette
a few cooked peas	

Simmer haddock in a little milk for 5 to 10 minutes. Drain, skin, remove bones, and flake. Heat in a little butter with peas and seasoning. Make an omelette in the usual way and fill with the fish mixture. Serve with quartered tomatoes. Serves 2–3.

BAKED PLAICE (FLOUNDER) AND PEACHES

1 large plaice (about 2 lb) filleted	salt and pepper
2 oz butter	a few grains of cayenne
1 lemon	peach halves, drained

Lightly grease a fireproof dish, and lay in the plaice fillets. Heat 1 oz butter in a small pan and add the grated rind and juice of half a lemon. Pour over the fillets, making sure the surface of the fish is well-coated. Dust with salt and pepper and a few grains of cayenne. Cook in oven—300°F—for 10 minutes. Heat remaining butter in a small pan till foaming. Add the peach halves which have been dried on a clean tea towel. Shake occasionally over moderate heat, allowing to caramelize slightly.

Remove plaice, without breaking, to a hot serving dish. Arrange peach halves on the dish. Place bouquets of watercress to garnish and lay lemon butterflies, made from remaining half of lemon, along edge of dish. Any juices left from baking should be poured over the fish. Serves 4–6.

FISH WITH WHITE GRAPES

4 fillets of sole, plaice or brill
6 oz white grapes
1 oz butter
2 tbs milk
¼ pt thick white sauce
2 egg yolks, beaten

Lay fillets out flat. Place a few white grapes, which have been halved and pipped, on each fillet. Fold into three. Place in an ovenproof dish with butter and milk and poach gently in the oven, about 325°F, for 12 to 15 minutes. Do not allow the liquid to do more than barely simmer.

When fish is tender, take up carefully and keep warm. Meanwhile, make a thick white sauce in the usual way, adding any fish liquid. When cooked, add the beaten egg yolks off the heat and stir briskly. Return to heat to thicken up. Pour a little sauce over each fillet and garnish with halved grapes. Serve with plain boiled potatoes. Serves 4.

TURBOT IN CHIVE BUTTER

4 5–6 oz turbot steaks
2 oz melted butter
1 tbs lemon juice
1 tsp chopped chives
salt and pepper

Brush the fish with half the butter and sprinle with lemon juice. Arrange in a greased shallow baking dish and cover with foil. Bake for 30 minutes at about 350°F or until the fish flakes easily with a fork.

Combine the rest of the butter with chopped chives and seasoning and heat slightly.

Arrange the fish on a serving platter and pour the warm herb butter over them. Garnish with parsley and slices of lemon. Serves 4.

COMPARATIVE CALORIE COUNT OF AN AVERAGE SERVING OF MEAT AND FISH

Beef, roast	210	Fresh haddock	115
Ham	320	Smoked haddock	120
Lamb	300	Halibut	140
Pork	360	Hake	90
Sausages (2 oz.)	145	Crab (2 oz)	75
Tongue	290	Herring	190
Liver	160	Mackerel	90
Corned beef	280	Plaice (Flounder)	90
Chicken	165	Lobster	65
Duck	190	Cod fillets	95
Turkey	185	Prawns	55
Heart	265	Herring	190
Mutton	300	Salmon	155

Breathe Deeper—Live Longer

WHEN YOU arrive at the seashore, almost the first thing you do is to take a deep, deep breath and then expel it forcibly with a satisfied: "Aaaah!"

Nobody has to tell you to breathe deeply. You just can't help it. "Breathe that wonderful air!" you exclaim: "It smells of ozone, it smells of the sea." You inhale, sending oxygen coursing through your body, renewing every part of it, pushing out the dead, stale, carbon monoxide- and dioxide-laden air of the city.

There is a Yoga saying that we have only just so many breaths allotted to us in a life span: if we take them slowly they will last that much longer and we shall live to be that much older.

Breathing is about the most important conscious function of the body. Important, did I say? It's vital! Stop breathing and it makes no difference whether your diet or your exercise program or your rest and relaxation have been adequate. The only other function of the body that is equally important is the beating of our hearts and we can't do very much about that. While we live it's automatic.

Breathing is only partly instinctive. True, we don't order ourselves to take each breath as it comes along. But we can command bigger, deeper, more rhythmic, lifegiving breaths.

Every part of the body is benefited by this sort of breathing, even the mind. It isn't only because the brain as much as any other part of the body needs oxygen. There is something more. Deep, rhythmic breathing has a calming effect on the emotions. If you think this is far-fetched, consider the opposite condition: fear, anxiety, worry—all of these are accompanied by quick, shallow, tense breathing. People who suffer from chronic anxiety, often with no real reason (and there are a great many who do suffer from this free-floating worry which is waiting to pounce on anything which it can get its teeth into) always breathe with quick, superficial breaths. These do not aerate the blood sufficiently, and many of the distant parts of the body do not get the oxygen they require. Carbon dioxide will not be effectively expelled.

The converse is also true. The habit of deep, slow breathing, with a certain period of breath retension in between inhalation and exhalation, has the effect of producing peace of mind that nobody can believe until he has tried it for a period. All the same, if you are worried or tense and take time to imagine yourself arriving at the seashore, breathing rhythmically (four seconds—or heartbeats—to breathe in, four to hold and four to exhale) you will soon find yourself feeling much calmer. The idea of counting ten when you are angry would be even more effective if you counted twelve, breathing rhythmically as you do so. You'll find it impossible to answer roughly while you are holding your breath and when you've finished the count, you won't want to. If you still do, keep on deep-breathing until you are completely untensed.

Instinctive or automatic breathing takes in about twenty cubic inches of air. That wonderful life-giving breath that we inhale at the seashore can increase the volume to a hundred, or even a hundred and thirty, cubic inches of air. That breath gives you four or five times as much oxygen to refresh your blood; that holding of the breath and final exhalation digs out from the generally unused bottom section of your lungs all the stale poisonous fumes that have collected there. Chasing through the bloodstream the oxygen goes about its helpful way of repair and renewal and the waste matter of cell destruction will be removed with greater thoroughness.

Count how many breaths you take in a minute normally. The long-lived turtle takes only three and there is an old Sanskrit proverb which says that if you breathe well you will live long on earth. You may find you are taking as many as sixty breaths in a minute. Try cutting it down to six. Perhaps you only took thirty. Four is not too hard, especially if you watch the second hand of a clock: five seconds to breathe in, five to hold, five to exhale. Even if you only spend five minutes a day doing this your health will benefit enormously. So will your figure.

At home, that is. At the seashore you are probably doing it anyway. One reason, among the many, that swimming is so good for your health and your figure is because it teaches you breath control. While your head is underwater, you have to hold your breath. Because you know this, you breathe in very deeply so that you have enough breath to hold. When you surface, you expel the air from your lungs because they are bursting to get rid of it. Then you start the rhythm again. Surf riding has the same effect. As you wait for a wave, you breathe deeply. As you plunge into the wave, you must hold your breath and retain it until you reach shallow water.

A swimming teacher told me that a pupil who had regularly practised the breast stroke without ever putting her face in the water asked his advice about how she could swim in a different style which would help her lose weight. He made her practise breath control, putting her face under water for two long strokes. In three months she lost eighteen pounds.

"What do you do when your women pupils want to lose weight but retain their hair set?"

"There are a lot of those," he said. "It just requires them to take a little more conscious thought. If they breathe in for two slow strokes, hold the breath for two more, expel on the last two and do this regularly they will lose weight if they need to but, curiously, if they are underweight they will gain."

As we get older, lungs become less elastic, the rib cage grows rigid and loses its power to expand fully. Too little oxygen in the bloodstream means more waste matter—uric acid in one of these. Waste substances can cause headaches, backaches, over- or under-weight, stiff muscles and joints, hardened arteries.

The skeptics among you are probably already shaking your heads. Uric acid? We-ell—maybe. But breathing can't possibly have any effect on living longer—as to weight control—utter nonsense!

It's not, you know. That five minutes of deep breathing —ten would be better—cleanses and stimulates the bloodstream, which in turn improves metabolism. A pepped-up metabolism will turn fat deposits into body fuel, and they can be used up for energy. This will reduce weight and expand years all in one go. Not in a day, of course, but in time.

A metabolism which works too fast is also at fault. This is usually found in a person who is tense, overactive, nervous, suffers from insomnia.

Breath control helps here, too, whether during swimming or by timed rhythmic breathing—and also in breath-controlled exercises. Nervousness—well, you know if you are going to make a speech and you feel scared, what do you do? Instinctively take a few deep breaths. If you are tense and wakeful you should try the same thing. Feel your pulse —maybe it is racing, but it is your pulse so use it. Lie on your back, hold the pulse of your left hand with the fingers of your right (or vice versa, if you'd rather). Breathe in for ten pulse beats, hold for ten, exhale for ten. Don't strain. If ten is too many, try five—but keep the equal rhythm between in, hold, out. Probably you find that when you are actually at the sea you won't need to do this, you will sleep well anyway. You have been swimming and exercising on the beach, you have breathed deeply, held your breath while swimming. Your bloodstream is cleaned out and purified by the good fresh air. Back at home it isn't so easy. But even the impure air of cities contains more oxygen than the used-up air of your lungs. Breathe yourself to sleep at night. Do some breathing exercises first thing in the morning (*see the end of this chapter*). And if, during the day you find you are involved in a tense situation, take a few deep breaths to calm down those stomach butterflies. It's better than any tranquillizer.

The free-floating anxiety which, as we said, is so prevalent in today's high-tension, high-speed life is almost always relieved by a week or two at the seashore. Why? Because it is not only easy to relax at the beach, it is almost impossible not to.

Beaches have a special fascination. Can you imagine any other place where you could find every inch of territory taken up by people lying around relaxed and almost nude, and having the time of their lives? A beach is synonymous with a holiday, and there is no doubt which comes first.

Children love sand—and it is sand, not the sea, that they cherish. They don't care so much for pebbly or rocky beaches (though the small pools in rocks are sometimes appealing). But they prefer sand that can be moved from here to there and which they can make into a mountain or a lake, a castle, a house or a fort. If your child wants to use you as the corner stone of his castle, encourage him. As we say in our slimming chapter, to lie covered from toe to neck in dry sand is as good as a Turkish bath and will draw a great number of impurities out of your system—things like uric acid, cholesterol, toxic poisonings which the sweat glands, given encouragement, are capable of throwing off. Of course, you can lie in the sun, or exercise and also sweat out impurities but evaporation causes many of the toxins drawn out by sweat to be reabsorbed whereas the sand retains them. You will emerge free from all those small aches and pains caused by uric acid and other acid products that tend to settle down uncomfortably in your muscles and joints.

If the sand happens to be wet you probably won't want to stay in so long. In this case the traffic will be going the other way. You won't excrete poisons, you will take on the benefits from the seawater still in the sand: the plankton, rich with life- and health-giving organisms from the sea. Their vitality will enable them to seep into your skin and act as a tonic. The minerals in the seawater are also all there for your skin's taking. You will get a vitalized mineral pack which will leave you exhilarated and filled with surging energy.

As well, a sand bath, wet or dry, will give you a rare combination of complete relaxation—the whisper of waves on the shore, the cooling breeze on your face—and stimulation. Your worries, along with your aches and pains, will all be drained away.

Twice a day the tide sweeps in, washing away every trace

of human occupation. The tides takes but it often leaves a bonus, a gift of some rare shell or polished glass jewel or a lovely piece of gnarled driftwood. Perhaps because I spent so much of my rather solitary childhood on a beach, I early became a scavenger. I called it treasure hunting then. I looked for shells large enough to be held to the ear. Inside these shells was the sea's roar. I looked for pretty seaweed and the skeletons of tiny animals or something tthat might have come from a wreck.

On the wide empty beaches of my childhood the retreating sea left miles and miles of firm sand. Overhead there were the shrieking, whirling seagulls. Beneath one's feet, the treasures and the taboos.

There were the jelly-fish-like party puddings, and the portuguese men-of-war, tourquoise blue balloons with long strings.

"Don't touch those, they sting."

As indeed they do, even after they are dead.

After storms weer sometimes mattresses, sodden, straw-filled, bursting at the seams.

"Don't touch that, a sailor may have died on it."

Well, this could have been true, too.

Cuttlefish. "What is this?" I ask.

"It's for canaries. We'll take it home for Dicky."

And although this was not its original purpose, it was true that Dicky liked it for beak-sharpening purposes.

Another time I found an oblong black bubble with points at each corner.

"That's a mermaid's purse," said the housemaid who was walking me out.

"May I pick it up?"

"Yes, but take your gloves off first, Miss Molly."

A mermaid's purse. There was no fairy gold in it except

in the idea itself. Much better than the reality I so carefully told my children on the New England beaches of their childhood. "It's the sack in which skates lay their eggs," I answered scientifically. That was the period when parents were told always to answer every question with the accurate truth if possible. With my grandchildren I shall return to fairy tales and Santa Claus.

Perhaps one of the very best reasons why people go to beaches for their holidays is that a beach is about the only place in the world where, work and problems forgotten—and indeed impossible—one can lie relaxed for hours with no sense of guilt. On a beach one exists like a plant or a flower and, like them, can use the sunshine to create a winter's supply of vitamin D. There is a rhythm in the wash of the water on the sand, of the predictable movement of the tide, of the beat of seabird's wings that is primeval. You empty yourself of time-tables, schedules, the endless pressures of the working year. You replace them with the calm of nothingness.

Sand, which is made of infinitesimal particles of rock, coral, shell, skeletons and many other substances, is washed by the tide, cleaned and replenished. The sea leaves behind, as well as tangible treasures, properties that are known to be healing to wounds, arthritis, bodily discomforts of many sorts. The surge of sand in the surf, beating on your legs, is beneficial to cramp. Sand is saturated with vitamin- and mineral-giving benefits; it is a first-class tonic healer—for the body—but also for the mind, the spirit, the soul, whatever you like to call the special something in your body that is you.

And perhaps, if you work at it a little, you can capture to bring home with you not only the physical benefits of sea, sand and sun but some of the peace of mind which these engender. If you lie, wakeful, tense, overwrought, cast your mind back and transfer your body from your bed at home to the warm sunny beach. Feel all your muscles relax as you sink into the sand. Breathe deeply of the ozone-laden air; watch the small sailboats bobbing on the waves and the sea-birds circling round them. Try to recapture in imagination the serenity of that scene. And sleep.

Ozone is a form of oxygen. It is antiseptic and destroys bacteria. Oxygen when exposed to ultra-violet rays forms ozone. Because of its disinfecting powers some cities—Paris, Philadelphia—use it as a disinfectant for water instead of chlorine. It can be produced by passing an electric current through oxygen or air. There are machines for doing this which if you have one in a bedroom, say, helps asthma sufferers and probably prevents colds. Ozone is also used in some air-conditioning systems.

At the beach it is there for you to breathe, and its odor is what encourages you to take those wonderfully beneficial deep breaths. Because ozone, if it penetrates skin, produces ultraviolet radiation at different depths of the tissue, it activates the circulation of the various depths of skin and helps to eliminate waste products. The effect of skin oxidation which comes naturally at the beach can be produced, artificially, by machines also.

BREATHING EXERCISES FOR THE BEACH OR THE HOME

People have been breathing ever since there have been people. Thousands of years ago wise men realized its importance and thought of ways that people could improve their breathing. In India it became part of their religion: they believed—and many still do—that in breathing they could draw some vital spiritual essence of life from the air.

They considered the breath of life highly significant for maintaining health and warding off disease, as well as for putting them in tune with the infinite. Because the shape of our lungs hasn't changed in thousands of years, breathing exercises that we do today are much the same as those done with religious fervor by the wise men of the Orient. You may not believe that there is any potential primeval force in the atmosphere. The air we breathe is nevertheless lifegiving. We might as well get as much of it as we can.

Nature, or whoever, creates a natural reflex movement in us when, air-starved, we come to the pure air of the beach. This same nature also causes instinctive shallow breathing where the air is scarce, smoke-laden, used up by too many people breathing it—in a cinema, a pub, a political rally. She (he or it) is protecting us from getting too much of the nasty polluted atmosphere into our lungs. In a thick smog one almost tries not to breathe at all. So, while it may not be easy, try to find the purest atmosphere you can in which to do your breathing exercises.

Shallow, smog-type breathing uses only the very uppermost part of the lungs. When the diaphragm is filled with air or rather expanded by the air in the lungs, this is better. To get to the depths of the lungs where pockets of foul fumes still congregate, the abdomen has to be expanded also. In breathing out, from a deep, abdominal breath, the first movement is to draw in the abdomen and press the air upward and out through the top of the lungs and the mouth. Because our noses have a filtering system of little hairs to catch germs before they can penetrate into the lungs, it is always best to breathe in through the nose. And because we want to expel as much used-up air as possible when we exhale, it is better to breathe out through the mouth.

So start by breathing out, trying to clear the lungs of

all the used-up air. To help you do this start by putting your hands on your abdomen, fingers spread out like that advertisement for a girdle, and press in, just like the ad. Start your intake by pushing your fingers away, not only with your muscles but also with the force of your inhalation. When these are pressed out as far as possible, move up to the diaphragm and expand the rib cage. Lastly, to get that extra little bit of air raise the shoulders slightly and complete the intake.

The balloon of your lungs is now full. Let the air out as if you had let go of the balloon. The air, of course, escapes through the mouth.

When you have learned to do this rhythmically and completely, breathe in to a count, hold for the same count, breathe out to the same also. It can be 4-4-4 or 7-7-7 as long as it is rhythmic.

Raising the arms above the head also helps you to fill your lungs. First, as you breathe in fully raise your arms sideways and place the palms together above your head. As you hold your breath bend from the waist sideways, left then right, left then right again. Exhale as you lower your arms. If at first you can only hold for one bend each side don't force it. In time you will manage three or four bends to one hold. Repeat this same exercise bending forward and backward, then twisting from the waist to the left then the right, then circling from the waist clockwise then counterclockwise. Remember to fill the lungs fully with each inhalation and to draw in the abdomen and press out every last bit of air with each exhalation.

A similar exercise which is a wonderful spine stretcher is done by raising the arms sideways, clasping the fingers, turning the clasped hands upward and pressing upward as hard as you can while holding the breath. Push the stars away from you.

Again, breathe in as you place your hand together in front of your chest, prayerwise. Press the palms together as you hold the breath. Bring them over your head and down to your side as you exhale.

Stand upright and clasp your hands behind your back. As you breathe in, use the weight of your clasped hands to pull your head backward. Lean over as far as you comfortably can. Hold for five counts and eventually for ten. Keeping the hands clasped behind come forward as you exhale completely. The head should come as near as possible to the knees with spine relaxed but knees straight.

Most breathing exercise routines that we do nowadays are derived in some part from Yoga. The Yoga religion places great stress on physical fitness, control of the body and deep, curative breathing. There is one ancient roundelay exercise in which breathing plays a strong part which, hundreds of years ago, must have been a religious practice since it is called the Sun Prayer. It is not a Yoga exercise but it does come from India.

It is quite hard to do in the beginning because it involves timing and breathing. I learned to do it by practising on the beach and now I pretend my rug is fresh, sea-washed sand. You can do the roundelay once, twice or three times—twenty if you could make it; I couldn't for many weeks. The last posture of one round is the first of the next. You can do it first thing in the morning, last thing at night, or any time in between. The round is said to use every muscle in your body and teaches you to breathe fully. Some people say that if you did it regularly you should never need another exercise. But I have so many exercises that I enjoy and feel are beneficial that I like to do these, at least some of them, every day, too.

Wear as little as possible—nothing if you do it in your own room but a swim suit or bikini on the beach.

Make a mark on the sand, or on the rug or towel: always, from the second to the ninth movement, keep your hands rooted to this spot. After you have tried out the exercise for a few times with the book try doing it in your mind only, remembering each movement and just where to breathe in and out until you know the routine by heart and you don't have to use the book any more. This takes patience and time—probably at least a week or even two so don't give up. I am afraid I did the first time. But after a few days I realized that I was missing out on an experience which could, if I really persisted, change my whole way of life. After doing them for a couple of months I lost all tendency to rheumatic or pre-arthritic pains, people remarked that I looked younger and, at exactly the same weight, I measured one inch less on the waist, one and a half on the stomach, and one and a quarter on the buttocks. Muscle weighs heavier but measures less than fat which accounts for the fact that I look and am a smaller size without weighing any less. My spine is stronger, a tendency to weakness and sometimes no longer feel the strain when I go downstairs. A friend of mine who suffered from constipation found this completely relieved. For this reason, and because the exercises help the skin excrete toxins, her complexion was enormously improved. An asthma sufferer, too, was greatly helped. With asthma it is exhaling that is the problem. Asthmatics may need the sort of training in exhalation that this exercise gives.

Position One is the same as position ten and is the first position of the next round, remember.

Place hands in a praying position in front of the chest. Stand erect, spine straight, feet firmly placed with weight on the outside of the foot, toes gripping the ground. Breathe deeply until your lungs are filled; at the same time stretching upward until every muscle of your body feels taut.

Position Two. Breathe out as you drop hands to the floor, fingers pointing slightly in, the ball of the thumbs opposite your feet. Throw your head toward your knees, which should be straight—but probably won't be at first. Try to aim at getting them as straight as possible.

Position Three. Breathe in as you drop the left knee to the ground. Keeping hands rooted press the right leg into your body. You are in the same position as a runner about to start a race.

Position Four. Still holding breath, raise body and move forward foot, the right, to join the left, your body forming an inverted V. In time you will be able to put your heels to the ground but don't force it.

Position Five. Keeping hands rooted, drop flat on the floor while exhaling. Press chin against chest, touching the ground with forehead, chest, knees and toes but keeping hips and abdomen elevated as high as possible. This squeezes the fat off the stomach and prevents the neck from developing a crêpey, hen's-throat look.

Position Six. Inhale as your straighten arms, curving spine and looking up to the ceiling. The arms take the weight, the throat muscles are stretched.

Position Seven. Holding breath, return to position four, the inverted V.

Position Eight. Holding breath, drop the right knee to the ground, pressing the left leg into your body. This is the same as position three except the reverse legs and different breathing.

Position Nine. Exhale, then same as position two.

Position Ten or one of next cycle. Breathe in.

Experts can do a complete round, and of course expertly, in seconds. A beginner takes much longer to complete it correctly. It does not matter. Do it as well as you can, for as many rounds as you can, taking ten minutes twice a day, morning and night. At night it helps promote healthful sleep.

Once you have learned to do the cycle correctly and automatically, even if you take as much as a minute, you will begin to get real enjoyment out of it. The benefits start even sooner.

Try to overcome any initial discouragement, stiffness, feelings of inadequacy and you will end up by feeling as healthy, every day of the year, as you do after two weeks at the seashore.

Slim the Mermaid Way

ABOUT NINE-TENTHS of the people who read this book wish they were a different shape. Slimmer, for example. So it seemed like a good idea to have a complete chapter on the subject of slimming. Those lucky people with an inner thermostat which roars up every time they consume, say, a pound of chocolates, burning it right up so that not even an ounce nestles in the wrong place, can just skip it.

Mermaids are always shown with gorgeous figures. How do they get them?

Well, swimming has a lot to do with it, I imagine. Who ever heard of an overweight fish? Even the so-called fat fish—mackerel, herring, sardines, salmon, tuna—are only just nicely rounded. Swimming is one of the best slimming exercises you can do. So many areas of the body are used, and used without the effort caused by gravity, that rhythmic, co-ordinated movements are possible which stretch and contract every wayward muscle, causing it to shed painlessly its pound of flesh. Swimming makes for poise and flexibility, too.

Swimming is good in any sort of water but it is especially good in the sea because you are getting the benefit of the sea salts on your skin. All the same, if you live in a city and can only go to an indoor heated swimming pool during the winter months—say twice a week—go anyway. There are a number of fabulous slimming exercises that can be done in water. Water is weight-bearing but provides a natural resistance. This means that you can do an entirely different kind of exercise, and use a different set of muscles, than is possible on dry land where not only have you to bear your own weight but provide your own resistance. You will find the exercises in detail at the end of this chapter.

So mermaids are slim because they swim, because they frolic around and exercise in water. Also, they live on the produce of the sea. They must eat a good deal of seaweed, fish, shellfish, plankton and such. Well, there's nothing else, is there?

It would be just as well for us if we were in the same position. We terrafermaids have no selectivity about our food at all. Left to ourselves we will usually take too much of what is bad for us, too little of what is good and wind up weighing twice as much and being half as healthy as we should.

The convenient thermostat control about which we were talking, which helps burn everything that comes its way, works perfectly in animals—and probably in mermaids. In people, taste, habit, social duties, and just plain greed interfere. The trouble with people is that they often have eyes bigger than their stomachs—though not for very long, abdomens being the cozy little storehouse for fat they so often are.

One doctor named the thermostat of the appetite the Appestat. If it were working perfectly, with no interference from our minds, it would regulate the heat of the body to control hunger and we would never overeat. It works for the mermaid because she doesn't have a candy store or kitchen refrigerator to run to for a quick nibble; therefore she does not develop an addition to, say, milk chocolate bars or some other form of carbohydrate.

Carbohydrate addicts have much the same problem as alcoholics or drug addicts. They just get a craving and that's that. But there's also another thing. Their internal arrangements may not be able to utilize carbohydrate—those over-processed white sugars and starches—and instead of converting them to energy, they turn them into rolls of fat. Calorie for calorie, they may not be eating much more or any more than their thin friends. It is just that due to some faulty mechanism their inner thermostat won't turn itself up high enough to burn the carbohydrates.

It's a good alibi all right—and nearly half the energy of overweight people is used up in searching for reasons why they just can't help being overweight. The bird they say they eat like is all too often an ostrich. And in fact the alibi only works if there was nothing that could be done about it. Like the alcoholic, the carbohydrate addict will have to recognize the weakness: an inability to eat sweets and such without adding poundage.

There are, of course, other alibis. Heredity—you can't help being fat, all your ancestors were. Answer: their food habits for generations have been at fault—and indeed you may suffer for this because you may have inherited their cookbooks and their addiction.

Defective glands. Answer: Well, that depends what you mean or if you now what you mean. The metabolism, which controls the rate at which you convert food to energy, body tissues and heat is controlled by the thyroid gland, and this, as we have already discovered, is dependent on iodine, the sea mineral. So here again the mermaid has an edge on the landladies.

For a variety of reasons overweight is age-making. Take appearance to start with. Your fat friends, wagging their double chins, will warn you against reducing, saying that your face will get thin and haggard if you diet. Nothing, of course, could be further from the truth. It is heavy jowls rather than clean young bones which are likely to make you look older. If there is no need to buy a belt because there is no waist to wrap it round; if you buy your dresses in the stylish stouts rather than the junior misses, you are probably looking ten years older than you need—and this is particularly true if you actually *are* ten years older.

"For the older person," says one specialist in senior citizenship, "the number of calories in the diet must be cut down. The decrease in natural activity from the age of thirty-five to sixty calls for an annual reduction of fuel food. Even if a person is as active at sixty as at thirty, thirty-five per cent fewer calories are needed. If the number of calories in food is not cut down, the weight will increase, and disability and death will be hastened. Lean people live longer, remain young, active, healthy and vital longer. This is probably a life-long principle."

That is to say, you should start young to balance the outgoing of energy with the incoming of fuel. How can you tell? The scales. When you are expending more energy you can eat more without putting on weight. If you are sitting around doing very little you will have to cut down. That's the way the cookie crumbles or the prune wrinkles.

"It's all nonsense about eating and overweight," a friend of mine argued with me. "At home, at work, I watch my calories like a hawk" (does a hawk watch his calories?). "And I have a hard time keeping my weight on an even keel. But when I went on holiday I decided not to bother, to eat what I wanted and enjoy myself. And I came back two pounds lighter than when I went away."

"So where did you go?" I asked.

"To the most wonderful little fishing village on the

west coast of France. Gorgeous beach, swimming, dancing, fishing—the lot. In the morning we played rounders on the beach and then went swimming. We sailed and fished in the afternoon and danced every evening. I ate like a horse."

Well, it's true that some horses are getting fish meal and powdered seaweed in their trough these days. Still——

"Sounds to me," I said, "as if you had eaten more like a mermaid. Seafood, mostly, I suppose? The fish you caught —or bought?"

"Everything!" she enthused. "Sea trout, lobsters, fresh mackerel—how different they taste right out of the sea! And then we dug for shellfish and prised mussels off the rocks and cooked them all together with the white fish we caught. It made the most wonderful *bouillabaisse*. So it just shows! Calories don't count."

They do, of course, to some extent. But you don't eat calories. You eat a certain quantity of food which gives you a certain amount of energy and it is this which is measured in calories. My friend was, in fact, eating rather low-calorie food and using up a good deal of energy. So she lost weight.

"Well," I answered, "you were getting your proteins from seafood, one of the best possible sources, and one which is much lower in calories than any other first-class protein. It contains plenty of iodine which may have pepped up your thyroid gland and therefore your metabolism. Then think of all the exercise you took digging, fishing, sailing and, best of all, swimming. Swimming and slimming are practically synonymous. People who can live that kind of life all the year round never get fat. They are too busy catching their main meal, and using up a lot of energy doing so, to have time for between-meal snacks, or those cocktail canapés or TV lunches. The kind of fat you ate in your fish is the kind that does not put on weight like the solid sort from meat."

"How could that be?" she asked.

"Well, as nutrition expert, Adelle Davis explained it, some seemingly fat people are only waterlogged. Unsaturated fat—the kind you get in seafood as opposed to land meat—helps shed this excess water. Also, when the right kind of fat is insufficiently supplied, sugar is changed to fat in the body more rapidly than it should. The third reason is that this quick change makes the blood sugar plummet causing hunger pains and a sort of faint feeling which seems to call for something sweet and fattening. Finally, fats are more satisfying than sweets and take longer to digest, therefore keep you from being hungry longer."

She picked up the first of these arguments.

"Excess water doesn't really count, though, does it. I mean, they say if you lose two pounds in a Turkish bath you gain it all back when you drink some water."

"Sweating—as you do in a Turkish bath—or for that matter in a seaweed or sand bath—or playing a strenuous game—helps shed weight quite apart from speeding up metabolism. When you shed water through the pores, you also shed a certain amount of fatty substances, such as cholesterol. Also, if you do happen to be the kind of person who retains more water in the tissues than you need—your ankles swell up, for instance—it is a good thing to get rid of the excess."

"What did you mean—sand or seaweed baths?"

"You can't take a sand bath or a real seaweed bath anywhere but at the beach. For the first you just get someone to cover you all over from the neck down with dry sand and stay in it for about ten or fifteen minutes. The sand will make you sweat but it will absorb the sweat and you won't feel anything—I mean any discomfort."

"And seaweed?"

"At our beach house we bring seaweed from the seashore every day, partly for the garden—it's a wonderful fertilizer. But also to put in the bath. Seaweed, combined with hot water, draws all the excess fluid and toxic substances out through the pores—it's terrific for rheumatism as well as for slimming. You can get it ashore too, though, in a liquidized form. When a well-known beauty queen told me she added seaweed fertilizer—which is, in fact, liquidized seaweed—to her bath for slimming I asked her whether a plain hot bath wouldn't do just as well. She claimed that not only did the seaweed bath make her perspire much more than just plain hot water but that the effect went on working for some time afterwards. That's why I thought I'd experiment with the real thing."

"And it did the trick?"

"It did the trick all right but it wasn't very practical, not for most people and not for most of the year even for the few. So I tried to see if I could find something that wasn't quite such a problem to remove from the bath but which would have the same effect. I looked around until I found a liquid seaweed preparation specially for the bath—sea foliage in solution, it calls itself. You can also get bags of dried seaweed, soak them for fifteen minutes in boiling water and add the liquid to the bath. The bag comes in handy for a friction massage which completes the effect of drawing blood to the skin's surface and cleaning out the impurities that have been drawn out through the pores."

"Don't you get frightfully hot and uncomfortable?"

"Not if you sponge your face with cool water from

time to time—the water absorbs most of the sweat so you don't notice it. As the perspiration draws off into the water the sweat glands keep producing more and a good many toxic substances are excreted. You do know, of course, that just as much waste matter leaves the body by way of the skin as from the kidneys or bowels? Then the heat causes the capillary blood vessels to dilate, the blood circulates more freely through the body. The good minerals from the seaweed, especially iodine, then penetrate the skin, stimulate and disinfect it."

"I didn't think the skin could 'absorb', as you call it."

"You did, you know. If you cut yourself and painted iodine on the wound you would expect it to be absorbed and to contribute to the disinfecting and healing of the cut, wouldn't you?"

There's another type of seaweed bath preparation made in West Germany and called Algemarin. We wrote about this in our seaweed chapter earlier, but we repeat for the benefit of slimmers.

The seaweed has been "fixed" a little so that it turns the bath the color of a coral reef. This does nothing for the figure but is of great benefit to the soul. Its faint sea pine scent is an additional bonus—the natural seaweed sometimes does remind one a little of low tide.

Its bubbles have this effect, according to Dr. Kerr Russel in a paper entitled *Foam Therapy*—which was about foam in general but seems to apply to this in particular. "The bubbles of foam," he writes, "are a splendid insulating material, so the heat of the water is dammed up in the body, metabolism is stimulated, the oxygen intake increases, and perspiration occurs freely without any exhaustion because the hydrostatic pressure of foam consists of nine-tenths air and only one-tenth water. Tests show," he adds, "that the surface vessels dilate, causing the blood pressure to fall and the work of the heart to be considerably lessened."

Since these sea algae contain sixty or more of the vital elements of sea water, specially including sea salt with all its trace minerals, you are getting a restorative treatment while you slim. The nerves are soothed, any stiffness wears off, and the skin surface is stimulated.

I think it is probably quite untrue that fat people are jolly. Of course, some may be, just as some thin people are also. But it does seem to be true that fat people are optimists—at least as far as a slimming program goes. They believe, well anyway hope, or perhaps wishfully think, that something, someday, somewhere, will slim them overnight—or at worst in a week or a month. A pill, perhaps.

I suppose it could happen. Years ago they would certainly have decreed that the lady was for burning if she had suggested such witchcraft as treating pneumonia with mould off a mushroom; yet when scientists turned it into penicillin nobody said a word. For that matter, they were already using foxgloves for the heart, the bark of a tree for malaria, so possibly seaweed pills can do something about overweight. The Institute of Seaweed Research does not believe that swallowing seaweed is slimming but they do say that it is splendid for you in other ways. A slimming pill including fucus is made by two different health food manufacturers—maybe more—and is said to work on some people. These are probably those whose thyroid gland needed some extra iodine and, having got it, is able, by means known only to this clever little endocrine gland, to boost metabolism and thus get food burned up before it can be turned into fat. It won't work on those whose gland is already well supplied. Even Sir Alexander Fleming did not claim that his penicillin would cure the pneumonia you didn't have. But the thyroid gland is not always working as efficiently as it might even if it is not in a bad enough way to cause goiter. Your thermostat may need to be switched up a little so that it can use food more effectively than just storing it up as fat.

The French have found a way of using plankton for spot reducing. Furthermore, their produce is under the patronage, they state, of M. le Ministre de la Santé Publique. Actually they have two products: plankton soap and plankton lotion. The soap also contains marine algae. I've no idea why it works but their explanation is that the sea plants are *particulièrement agissants* and these infiltrate into the fatty tissues and neutralize the excess—and only in the area on which it is applied.

The whole subject of slimming is complicated by the fact that some things work on some people and not on others. But it is said to be true of everyone that a certain amount of energy—measured in calories if you like—is used up in the mere eating, that is, in the process of digestion which, when you go into it, is quite a complicated procedure. All that food has to be divided up and apportioned to its various tasks and turned into this and that. One slimming expert based his entire slimming program on the premise that a head of lettuce, say, is a plus food, providing about twenty-five calories of energy and using up thirty-five in its digestion. Protein uses up more calories in this way than either fat or carbohydrates. In addition, it is satisfying so that slimmers don't get hungry. The amino acids, which form protein, help the conversion of fats, sugars and other starches into useful ingredients for growth, repair and energy instead of allowing them to be stored up.

Any protein will do this. But since the protein of fish and especially shellfish is very much lower in caloric value than the protein of meat, while at the same time it uses up about the same number of calories in its digestion, it is sensible to eat as much fish as possible in place of meat on your slimming diet.

The type of food you choose to eat helps. In the long run the way to be slim, and remain slim, is to balance what you take in again what you put forth: if you eat more you must exercise more. An American doctor says: "The practice of overeating, of stuffing more fuel into the machine than is needed either for its maintenance or its functioning, is so widespread in the United States as to constitute a national vice. A moment's reflection will show how dangerous is the effect of overeating. The body is a machine designed to break down its own fuel, to burn it, to get rid of the waste products. When food intake is excessive and body cannot burn it fast enough. It becomes choked and poisoned by products of its own overloaded metabolism. Kidneys are overburdened. Great rolls of fat interfere with the movement of muscles and place an added burden on the heart, all of which can be corrected by the very simple expedient of balancing fuel intake against fuel requirements."

To be slim and stay that way, you have to be aware of what you are eating. Choose foods that are high in protein, minerals and vitamins and low in calories: seafood is all these. Watch your scales and if the needle goes over the desired mark, add exercise and subtract high-calorie, low-nutrition food (sugars, starches). It isn't only that you'll live longer, you'll also live longer looking younger, feeling healthier. It's worth it.

SLIMMING EXERCISES FOR THE BEACH AND
THE SWIMMING POOL

Run along the beach in two feet of water, raising the knees as high as you can. If you find two feet too deep, start with one. Of course the tide's flow necessarily alters the depth of the water as you run but that makes your canter all the more effective.

It is also wonderful exercise to walk on very soft sand. And try it on your knees, head held high, tummy tucked in. You won't get far but you will use up a lot of energy.

The breathing exercise in the last chapter, especially those you do when you are swimming, are invaluable figure proportioners.

Exercises in the sea or the pool—the best kind of pool, of course, is one where the water is filtered in from the sea, but a fresh-water swimming pool is better than nothing—are non-weight bearing and against resistance. The water bears your weight, as I said, in a way that air doesn't —you can't swim through air three feet from the ground. On the other hand, air offers no resistance to the free movements of arms and legs. Water does. It is this basic fact that makes water exercises completely different from air exercises. To take one example. If you stand upright, out of water, raise your leg slowly sideways, you are working against gravity and the muscles down the top of the leg, from hip to ankle, get the hard work. As you drop the leg with the aid of gravity you need do no work at all and no muscles have to put forth effort. When you do the same exercise in water, about three or four feet deep, the leg will float up to the surface with a minimum of effort but must be forced downward against the resistance of the water. You will therefore find yourself using the usually neglected muscles of the inside of the thighs—and these are muscles which one sees loose and flabby looking on quite young people.

1 Stand in water up to your neck, feet wide apart, arms outstretched, tummy taut. Twist at the waist, swinging the whole torso sideways. Take it slowly and deliberately consciously pushing the water away from you with your arms.

2 This is a similar exercise but clasp your hands together at chest level, elbows out. This time, as you twist from the waist, keep your head still, looking straight ahead, so that only the trunk and arms turn, pivoting on the neck above and the hips below. (And do this exercise on dry land also, concentrating your attention on the muscles at each side of the tummy, feeling them rubbing away their coating of fat.).

3. Skip on alternate feet, raising knees as high as possible.

4 At the depth of about four feet, run, raising knees. If there are not too many people in the pool, run right across from side to side. If there are, run on the spot.

5 Rise up on the tips of your toes. Margot Fonteyn style. The water will be your ballet shoes, keeping you from falling. If there is room, walk on ballet-toes across the pool, water at neck level, body pulled right up as if a cord was tied to your head.

6 At a depth of three feet do a Russian sword dance, shooting your feet out in front of you alternately.

7 Hold on to the side of the bath with the fingertips, elbows down, forearms resting on the side of the bath; kick alternate legs back as far as possible, vigorously.

8 Hold to the side of the bath with fingertips, stretch arms to full length, walk up the edge of the bath as far as

you can with straight legs. Hold at the highest point, walk down again.

9 Stand upright at the side of the pool depth about four feet. Let each leg float up sideways, then vigorously pull it down again so that your feet are together again. Repeat on the opposite side. This is the exercise which tightens up those flabby inner thigh muscles.

10 If nobody is using the springboard for diving on, jump up out of the water to grasp the sides as near the front as possible. Draw yourself out of the water, bending your elbows and knees (your knees as near to your chest as you can manage, then let go so that your spine stretches from the neck down. Repeat once. You will feel your body stretching tall and slim as the legs drop, but it will not be too hard on your arms as the water will take most of your weight.

11 At the beach: lie in the shallows where the waves will roll over you. Point your toes seaward and as the wave reaches you, raise your hips from the ground, bearing your weight on your arms. Arch your back and lean your head slightly backward. The surge of the waves stimulates circulation, which helps the system rid itself of unwanted fat.

In most of these exercise repetition is not the important thing. Do them as many times as you wish without tiring yourself. It is much more effective to hold the stretch for a few seconds at its furthest point and do the exercise once, than to do ten quick, jerky, flabby movements. In this way your muscles respond to the gentle pressure and will be a little more pliable and less resistant every day.

And, of course, there is no exercise which does more for the figure than swimming itself. An underwater massage, whether in the bath or the sea, a squeezing and a kneading of those little rolls of fat round the tummy, hips or thighs helps loosen them up so that the exercise can tighten up muscles, the stimulated circulation carries away excess fat. It all helps overweight and it is wonderful for the health, too.

And keep doing your Sun Prayer exercises when you come out of the water—or before you go in. Or, throughout the year, at home. You will gain and maintain good health, a whistlestop figure and a disposition which not only makes you feel happy but which sheds happiness around you.